The World
of the
Unborn

The World of the Unborn

Nurturing your child before birth

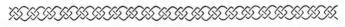

Leni Schwartz, Ph.D.

Preface by Gay Gaer Luce
Foreword by Don Creevy, M.D.

Richard Marek Publishers
New York

Library of Congress Cataloging in Publication Data

Schwartz, Leni.
    The world of the unborn.

    Bibliography: p.
    Includes index.
    1. Pregnancy—Psychological aspects. 2. Prenatal influences. 3. Prenatal care. 4. Parent and child. 5. Childbirth—Study and teaching. I. Title.
RG560.S4   618.2'4   80-17223
ISBN 0-399-90090-X

Grateful acknowledgment is made for permission to reprint material from the following works:

Poetics of Space, Gaston Bachelard, Beacon Press, 1969.

The Search for the Beloved by Nandor Fodor, Permission granted by University Books, Inc. 120 Enterprise Ave. Secaucus, New Jersey 07094.

Realms of the Human Unconscious by Stanislav Grof and Joan Halifax-Grof, Copyright © 1975 by Stanislav Grof and Joan Halifax-Grof, Reprinted by permission of Viking Penguin Inc.

Life Before Birth by Ashley Montagu, The New American Library, New York.

The Developing Human by Keith L. Moore, W.B. Saunders & Co. Copyright © 1979 by The New York Times Company. Reprinted by permission.

Love and Will by Rollo May, 1969. Reprinted by permission of W.W. Norton & Co. Inc.

Your Baby's Brain Before Birth by Mortimer G. Rosen M.D. and Lynn Rosen Ed. D. The New American Library, New York.

Broca's Brain by Carl Sagan, Copyright © 1979 Random House.

An article by Judith Thurman, Copyright MS. Magazine Corp. 1975. Reprinted with permission.

Garuda III: Dharmas Without Blame, Copyright © 1973 by Chögyam Trungpa. Reprinted by special arrangement with Shambala Publications, Inc., 1920 Thirteenth Street, Boulder, Colorado, 80302.

The Psychoanalytic Study of the Child, "Some Considerations of the Psychological Processes in Pregnancy," by Grete L. Bibring. International Universities Press, 1959.

Page 310 constitutes an extension of the copyright.

Acknowledgments

So much of my life's journey is represented in the creation of this book that it is impossible to list or even trace all those who have influenced it. So many have generously shared their time, their thinking and their hearts. Many advisors have become valued friends and many friends have been valued advisors. They have stimulated, challenged and nurtured me. In these pages, I can name but a few who have played direct and indirect roles in helping me and this project along. To all those who have been an integral part of my life and to those with whom I have only had brief but significant contact, I am deeply grateful.

I am particularly indebted to Dr. Stanislav Grof, for it is out of his creative perception and research that my work evolved. His sustaining friendship and encouragement of the work I began was continually supportive. It was my friend, Jill Kneerim, who helped me initiate and focus this book. Without her generosity of time and spirit, professional clarity and belief in it, this book would never have come to be. She helped me find my own voice as I struggled to express myself in a new and unfamiliar form.

The ideas and encouragement of my Ph.D. committee started me on my journey. I wish to thank Rita Arditti, Norris Clement, Joan Halifax, Gay Luce, Lockwood Rush and Dr. Harold Wise. They were challenging mentors. Harold Wise, joined by Richard Grossman, continued to influence my thinking as stimulating colleagues and close friends as we developed a model for "The Family Center" in New York. The support of the Benjamin Rosenthal Foundation made our year together possible. Joseph Campbell's vast knowledge of mythology and its relevance to the unfolding of life has been a source of inspiration and his friendship a wellspring of support.

Many widened my perspective of this subject through the generous sharing of themselves and their work. In particular, I want to express gratitude to Suzanne Arms, Raven Lang, Dr. Don Creevy, Dr. Milton Estes, Dr. Jeffrey Anderson, Sheila Kitzinger, Dr. Arthur Colman, Dianne Connelly, Libby Colman, Rollo May,

Jean Houston and Dr. James Herzog. I also want to offer thanks to Dr. Cliff Saron and Dr. Roger Walsh for their reading and constructive suggestions for Chapter II, and my appreciation to Judith Thomas and Amy Ameen for their help.

Most particularly, I wish to acknowledge the work of Barbara Riddle, who collaborated with me on the final draft of this book. Without her help in restructuring the unwieldy amount of material, it could not have been completed. I have appreciated her ideas, intelligence and skill.

The experience of pregnant parents is at the heart of this book. I'd like to express my gratitude to each member of the Birth Workshops for their active participation, to Maryallen Gessart and Charles Goodrich for their involvement and assistance in leading groups and to my friends, Eleanor Briggs and Hilary Harris, for their contribution of professional assistance with videotape and photographic documentation.

Many good friends have sustained me in this effort with their love, encouragement and ideas: Jacqueline Doyle through her insight into the nature of relationships and transition and her experience in leading groups. She was also always there when I wavered, as was Patricia Ellsberg, whose spirit and insight often kept me going, along with a whole group of wonderful people who have shared ideas and stood by me during these years of intense personal evolution. They have been dear friends, models, truthsayers. I feel blessed. Among them are Elizabeth Campbell, Dr. Len Duhl, Paul Gaer, Mary Kohler, John Kohler, John and Beth O'Neil, Brendan O'Regan, John Levy, Claire Merrill, John Parkinson, Natalie Rogers, Jeanne and Bill Ross, Frances Vaughn and June Wise.

Transforming this book into a reality was accomplished with the help of some special people—Joyce Engelson and Elaine Markson. Their enthusiasm for the project has been important to its completion. I am grateful to them both, as well as to Ursula Bender and Andre Schiffrin.

I thank everyone from the bottom of my heart.

*To my parents and to my children
with whom I have experienced
the process of birth most intimately. . . .*

Contents

Preface

This very personal book is a good preparation for giving birth and becoming included in the feelings and experiences of generations of parents. It is a guide to becoming a parent consciously and openly, and an admittance to the secrets—the feelings—that are rarely transmitted in this peculiar culture of ours. Many parents must have a feeling of "Oh, my God, what have I gotten into?" when they come into full awareness of the mysterious function they are fulfilling. It is out of their control. They have been willing pawns of forces well beyond rational understanding. And when a baby is securely on its way, they are the bridge, about to enter a uniquely binding relationship in which they will have to become the basis for that person's very survival, its significant teachers, the creators of an environment for emotional and spiritual growth. It is an amazing responsibility and process.

In pregnancy and dying we humans become aware of the intimacy between absolute and relative reality. Perhaps that is why we feel an awesome, inarticulable quality about these two processes. In one, the person journeys out of his small form into vastness. In the other, a mother becomes the vessel for the long journey from free and formless space into the shape and vicissitudes of a human infant. We recognize that these two processes are unique in our lives, and yet in this strange cultural period we act as if we take them for granted. We do not express our deepest feelings, our respect for the process of life. Instead, we often avoid the departing person, and give little real support or guidance (we tend to offer information or techniques instead) to the parents awaiting the arrival from inner space. So we often leave in isolation the very people who face life and death at their most imminent, at the crucial times when people need all the wisdom the race can offer them. Enhancing the cruelty of this isolation, most birthing and dying take place in the sterile environments of hospitals. At these significant hours, entering or leaving life, we are bathed more in efficiency than love, in antisepsis rather than reverence.

13

We have become trained to absorb our attention in practicality and to overlook the awesomeness of these processes until the experience is actually upon us. No wonder we have fears. No wonder we keep them to ourselves, even feel guilty about them. To whom can we honestly express our feelings?

Leni Schwartz and all the others who have taken birth seriously enough to alter this situation are initiators of a new trend toward making parenting and arrival on this planet a more conscious, joyous, and shared experience. Whatever affects the mother and father and the birth process must inevitably leave its imprint on the entire life of the child. Leni Schwartz, in her prebirth groups—for which the instructions are included here—is helping to set the stage for happier, more deeply experienced pregnancies and births, and thereby, we must assume, for saner babies and adults.

GAY GAER LUCE

Introduction

Embryo, fetus, unborn child—none of these words adequately conveys the nature of the being who, day by day, becomes more human on its journey to the outside world. We know that from the first moment after conception, the full human potential exists, waiting to be elicited and influenced. But no single word summons up the profound complexity of the future possibilities of this person in the womb—the "preborn" human being. If I were writing in a language with different rules, I would be at liberty to create a word that embodied the concept: the *becoming/human*, the *emergent/person*. Since English is my language, it will take all the words in this book to transmit to you my sense of the humanness of the child before birth, and also my feelings about how our experiences before birth are connected to our lives afterwards.

Truly, at the heart of this book is the unborn baby and the ways in which it is affected by the emotional life and daily rhythms of its parents, and then by the circumstances of its birth. Research that has accumulated over the last several decades has brought into being a new field, fetology, that honors this earliest period of human life and assesses the effects of everything in the unborn child's environment. Psychiatrist James Herzog, of Harvard Medical School, even suggests that a new field—the "psychoembryology of parenthood"—be given emphasis and integrated into studies of fetal embryology. With this term, Herzog is acknowledging the importance of the inner life of expectant mothers and fathers, and the role that these inner events play in affecting the parents' ability to bring into being and nurture a child.

Eight years ago, based on my growing understanding of the developmental implications of the pregnant year, I began to design pregnancy support groups for men and women who wanted to explore their feelings during the childbearing year, and begin to make an emotional connection to their not-yet-born children. In a sense, we were engaging in a "prenatal bonding" ritual; although we could not hold and touch the babies, we could speak to them, fantasize about them and prepare ourselves for the next stage by making the transition to familyhood on a gradual basis rather than in one sudden plunge after labor and delivery.

As this book documents, these groups had enormous value for those who participated. Step by step, I describe our early attempts to develop these workshops, and I suggest specific ways in which you might make these groups a reality in your own community. Finally, I offer my vision of a birth center that would provide an environment where babies could be born, and families could evolve, in harmony with the parents' emotional needs and with the highest regard for the health and well-being of their baby.

Prologue

It was the first month of one of my workshops for pregnant couples. Women and men who were moving through the changes of pregnancy and preparing themselves to becoming parents gathered together once a week for four months, and, under my guidance, were seeking answers to questions that had never occurred to them before.

We began the first session with an exercise designed to create an awareness that the developing baby was, in fact, a person who could be communicated with emotionally and physically:

All of you are here as couples, partners in a joint venture—but actually, there's a third person here with you. Over the next months we're going to focus on how we can bring that third person into each of your lives in a daily way . . . how you can become a family and discover what it means to be consciously sensing yourself as one of the three parts of the whole, even before the actual birth of your child.

To focus your awareness on the threesome you are becoming, I'd like to start this evening with an exercise that will help us to be mindfully aware of the unseen participants in this workshop, the persons with whom we'll be developing an intimate relationship during the coming months.

Concentrate on yourself as couples, and as a family . . . on two becoming three. . . . Pay attention to your own breathing and the flow of your joint breathing as it enters your body . . . as it fills your heart, moves through the body, through your arms and legs and out again into the room, exhaling your breath out and inhaling it in again, adjusting the rhythm of your breathing to that of your partner's. And again inhale, be aware of your environment, focus on moving your breath through your body into your heart and into the heart of your baby. . . .

No one in the room stirred, eyes were closed, fingers were entwined. It appeared that each threesome was wrapped in attentive meditation and visualization as they sat opposite each other, knees touching.

Allow your breath to flow freely from father to mother and child. Visualize the baby's environment inside the water-filled womb. . . . Think about the baby's experience of its environment, its sense of you and the world beyond you. Think about what you are communicating right this minute to the responsive being who is forming in the womb, a baby that you have created. Think about yourself and what you feel as mother, as father, as a woman, as a man. . . . Stay in touch with yourselves as a threesome, as a family. . . . When you are ready, open your eyes slowly and gaze at each other. Take time to be with each other silently, and when you are ready, each of you individually write a dialogue with the baby.

There was stillness; there were no restless movements. Not even Barbara stirred, despite the pressure of her full belly pushed tight against her breasts. Jim's hands held hers, resting on the shelf created by the swollen womb. Karin and Andy sat on the floor, facing each other, no longer quite so erect, leaning towards each other as they remained in meditation. Jim opened his eyes and watched Barbara in her reverie, her eyes still closed. Slowly he raised her left hand to his lips. She opened her eyes to his touch, his head bent over his kiss. She smiled.

Everyone began to write. Twenty minutes later, we shared our dialogues. The fathers began. Andy said:

* * *

It's really hard to relate to you, since I can't see you or
feel you. It's hard to believe in the reality of you living
in the womb or even in my connection to you. Did I
really have a part in conceiving you? My head tells me
that's true, but my psyche is struggling to understand
my part in it.

Jim wrote, "If I were you, kid, I'd want to get out of there."
Barbara was furious. It never occurred to her that her baby
wasn't happy in the environment she was providing. She felt put
down as Jim argued that nine months was a long time to be
trapped in that space.

Ed asked me what I was driving at in suggesting such a
dialogue.

Do you really believe we can affect the baby in the
womb, by loving it, for instance? How can I influence
the baby in my wife's belly?

Although he admitted he was surprised by his sense of contact
with the baby, and had written three pages of dialogue, he was
now rationalizing those feelings away as he pressed for evidence.
When I suggested that he did indeed affect his wife's emotions
each day, which then directly influenced the baby's uterine existence, he laughingly denied that he had any sway over his wife.

"Anyway," said Ed, "what makes you think there is consciousness in the womb?"

He had raised one of the most fundamental questions of the
workshop.

In this book, I trace the events in my life that led to my
interest in this question and why I think the subject has such
far-reaching implications for each of us. My research and my
personal explorations have convinced me that our conscious lives
begin in the womb. Accepting this idea can lead one in two

seemingly opposite, but complementary, directions. One can learn more about one's own birth and gestation, seeking clues to how one's own inner psychology and temperament may have been shaped by very early experience. Others may concentrate on modifying current practices in regard to pregnancy and childbearing to make these periods as beneficial as possible to baby and parents in light of new findings in the field of fetal development. It seems to me that the possibilities for individual growth and cultural change are enormous. I offer this book as a beginning tool for those who wish to begin—or continue—this quest. In particular, it may be used as a guide to forming support groups for men and women who are preparing for parenthood.

The exercise in communicating with the baby, described above, is one that I developed during a series of four-month-long workshops that I led in New York and San Francisco during the mid-70s. Four or five couples participated in each workshop during the course of their pregnant year, exploring with me the psychological and social aspects of pregnancy as they affected the emerging families.

The chapters that follow elaborate on the problems and solutions that emerged as I continued to lead workshops for pregnant couples. During this period it was my constant hope that these weekly gatherings would be joyful, celebratory occasions for examining and understanding the potentially stressful changes of the pregnant year, in order that it might be the fully transformational period that nature seems to have designed.

As an artist and designer, I had originally been concerned with creating beautiful physical environments for *birth*, but when I begin to perceive the impact that the prenatal environment had, I realized that I needed to consider the *entire* environment of birth. Parents should be able to anticipate and shape not only the physical/medical aspects of their baby's birth, but the emotional/spiritual/social ones as well. How I came to create and lead these workshops is itself a story of growth and development—my own, as I moved from one cycle in my life to another, undergoing radical transformations that made me especially sensitive to the experiences of the men and women in my groups during the transitional crisis of pregnancy.

How Did the Workshops Come to Be?

For most of my life, I have been fascinated by designing and planning spaces in which people live and work. Even as an adolescent, in hopes of effecting changes in my family's life together, I continually rearranged the furniture to create new environments. Toes and shins were continually at risk for any unsuspecting member of the family who came into the darkened room unaware that I had rerouted the old familiar pathway. Since then I have become an interior designer and a painter. For twenty years, I have collaborated with architects and individuals in designing the spaces in which people live.

Gradually, I began to question my status as an "expert" to whom people willingly gave the power to make decisions about the environment in which they worked, played and loved. In an effort to reverse this procedure, I found myself spending more and more time involving others in understanding their own needs and choices. I moved from the role of professional designer to explorer to student, and initiated a course of personal study, starting with a course in environmental psychology offered by the City University of New York.

My whole life focus began to shift. In 1971 I entered a Ph.D. program that started out with a broad environmental focus and then became dramatically centered on my concept of "the environment of birth." This new emphasis in my life and in my work emerged from an experience whose meaning and ramifications I am still in the process of understanding. This book is an exploration of that experience and how I have attempted to apply the insights I gained from it in ways that would be useful to others.

What was this profound experience? I believe it was none other than the guided "reenactment" of my own birth, in a manner that changed many of my assumptions about how and why we become who we are, why we behave the way we do, to what extent we can shape our own lives. Specifically, I now see life in the womb, and birth, as a continuum of processes that affect us throughout our entire lives.

Therefore, this book is about not only the birth process, it is about life and the integration of all our experience. The process of birth has become for me a metaphor for how the universe is patterned, the part standing for the whole—an "ordinary" process which allows us to perceive the extraordinary dimensions of life. This book is about the constant challenge to integrate change into continuity, to see patterns of growth and renewal in all aspects of our lives—not just our first beginnings—to understand how we and the universe are interdependent.

The World of the Unborn

Foreword

The last several decades have seen a distillation in the Western world of the knowledge and experience of generations of women, midwives, and physicians regarding childbirth. Read, Lamaze, Bradley and their advocates have returned to women the tools and confidence with which to give birth in a safe, wholly satisfying way. Leboyer, Klaus and Kennell have heightened our awareness of the extreme sensitivity of the newborn to its physical and psychological environments. Suzanne Arms has shown women that the right to self-determination in pregnancy and birth is theirs, despite a long history and strong tradition of male-dominated, technologically oriented obstetrical care. Sheila Kitzinger has described in universal terms the feelings of women about childbearing and the psychological impact of becoming a mother.

Now Leni Schwartz, in this wonderfully readable and practical book, places a new focus on the couple and their psychological and physical environment during the childbearing year. She draws upon the traditional psychiatry of Jung and Freud as well as the new expressions of personal freedom and fulfillment of the many visionaries in the human potential movement. She shows us how the expectant couple may work together, with other couples and with health professionals to develop feelings of confidence and control over their internal and external environments. This process is critically important to the successful creation and nurturing of a new person and a new family.

Her acute observations and useful techniques add yet another dimension to society's care of its developing families, and should be shared by physicians, midwives, childbirth educators and all those who have an interest in the health and welfare of our new babies and their parents.

This book has enriched my perception and will have a pro-

25

found impact on the care I give to the childbearing woman and her family.

—Don C. Creevy, M.D.
Obstetrician/Gynecologist
Stanford University
School of Medicine,
Stanford, California

I

What Is Birth?
When Does Being Born Begin?

Life is a continuity which does not begin at birth; it is split up by birth. The result of this splitting up is prenatal amnesia, but there is also an unconscious persistent effort to reestablish the lost continuity by annulling the trauma of birth.

Nandor Fodor,
Search for the Beloved

Birth is not a beginning . . . the true beginning is at conception. Nor is birth an ending. It is more nearly a bridge between two stages of life, and although the bridge is not a long one, a child crosses it slowly, so that his body may be ready when he steps off at the far end.

Ashley Montagu,
Life Before Birth

Reliving My Birth

In the fall of 1971, I attended a lecture by Dr. Stanislav Grof, a renowned research psychiatrist. In his early forties, outwardly conservative-looking in his suit and tie, as he talked the depth and originality of his thinking became increasingly apparent. He presented a map of the complex levels of human consciousness manifested by his patients during the many years of his research with LSD therapy. Originally trained as a traditional Freudian psychoanalyst, Grof had conducted LSD research in his native Czechoslovakia, and since 1967 had been working in the United States by special invitation of the Maryland Psychiatric Research Institute. He spoke of psychedelic drugs and particularly LSD, as tools that, properly used, could enable one to study psychic material that is buried in the deepest layers of the unconscious and is usually inaccessible to less dynamic techniques.

His theoretical framework for understanding the levels and dimensions of consciousness was derived from an analysis of material culled from three thousand sessions conducted over the course of twenty years. All patients apparently moved through similar levels during their LSD sessions: first through the individual psychological levels of their experience—birth, childhood, adulthood—and then "spontaneously into experiential realms

29

that have been described through the millennia as occurring in various schools of the mystical tradition, temple mysteries and rites of passage in many ancient and pretechnological cultures of the world. The most common, as well as the most important, of these phenomena were experiences of death and rebirth, followed by feelings of cosmic unity."

One of the major categories of psychedelic experience observed by Grof is unquestionably connected to the first and possibly most traumatic event of our lives: birth. Several times, in the course of long-term LSD psychotherapy, most patients experience a remarkable, harrowing reenactment of the unexpectedly traumatic nature of the birth process: the insistent pulsation of the womb's contractions, the compressing sensations of the squeeze through the narrow opening, the cranial pressure, the rough handling by attendants and the profound shock of the sudden expulsion into the extrauterine world. Subjects frequently assume postures and move in complex sequences that resemble those of a baby at various stages of delivery. Grof, and other therapists who utilize a range of techniques that evoke powerful sensations related to the birth process, found that most participants later recounted the experience in incredulous language; it seems to be universally difficult to accept the idea of such preverbal memory. Paradoxically, subjects remain convinced that they have experienced reenactments of their births.

Dr. Grof's observations suggested that the memory of our own birth may lie within each of us and can, under the right conditions, be evoked and "reexperienced." Extremely stimulated by the implications of his findings, I approached Dr. Grof after his talk and asked if we could meet again to discuss his research. We met the next day. I learned more about his work and told him about my own interests and concerns. His lecture had revived an earlier interest of mine in taking LSD under clinically controlled conditions where I might feel free to be open to the insights released by the drug. I was acutely conscious of the importance of having a psychologically and medically trained guide for my journey into such an unexpected part of myself. When I learned of the three research programs that he was supervising at the Maryland

Psychiatric Research Institute in Baltimore, I volunteered for one that was to study the experience of artists, writers, theologians and psychologists.

Through these various programs, Grof was continuing his long-term process of mapping the levels of the human unconscious. His recent book presents a careful description of his philosophy, clinical approach and findings (see Bibliography). The Baltimore clinic was one of the last remaining clinics in the U.S. in which approved and funded LSD research was taking place. It appeared that if I was accepted into the program, I would have an experience which I had first sought ten years earlier.

For more than a decade I had been intrigued by the idea of "altering" my consciousness in order to explore hidden layers of my unconscious.

Why was I intrigued? As a designer, I was interested in discovering how we develop our preferences and tastes in art and music, or why we choose to have certain shapes or colors in our homes. Grof's work implied that we are influenced very early on, possibly even in the womb, and that we remember our earliest experience in some as yet unknown way. Like most of us, I was—and am—searching for a way of understanding and expressing the core of self that is uniquely me. For me, LSD therapy with Grof promised to be a powerful way of reaching these deeper levels.

Although I was pleased to be considered for the Baltimore project, I was nevertheless quite scared at the prospect of opening up to such an unknown experience. I went through the interviewing and psychological testing procedures which were an integral part of his research study and was approved for the program. I was considered a mature, psychologically healthy subject: married for twenty-three years, mother of three grown children, a professional artist and designer. A date was set for my first session.

The afternoon before the scheduled session, Grof and I talked about what I might expect from the next day's journey. He described the procedure, the time sequence (eight to twelve hours) and showed me the environment in which it would take place. He explained to me that I would lie down on a couch, use eye shades, headphones and music and be encouraged to remain in a reclining position. "We have found," he said, "that these procedures help people focus on the internal phenomena that are unfolding, and prevent external distraction. Music is played throughout the session and is an integral part of the experience. The headphones intensify and deepen the experience." He suggested I choose from the library of records a selection of my favorites that I felt would evoke a range of emotional responses from me. During the session, he continued, he preferred to keep verbal communication to a minimum so that conversation would not intrude on my experience, but he assured me that he would be there and would be aware of my needs. He reviewed the nature of the states of consciousness that the psychedelic experience may produce. He asked questions: Was I nervous? How was I feeling? Was there anything in particular that I was concerned about? We talked about the history and the issues I was confronting in the life transition I was moving through. We discussed my longings and fears and expectations and the wide swings of elation and depression that I had been experiencing recently—not unlike the emotional ups and downs of the pregnant state. Indeed, I was pregnant with a new self.

There was much change occurring in my life, some of it reflecting the sweeping social upheaval that was affecting couples everywhere, some of it unique to the circumstances of my life and of my need to develop my individuality. I was moving into another cycle. The nurturing role, which had been a paramount one for many years, was being phased out: my children—twenty-two, twenty and eighteen—were grown up and living away from home. Maternal and household concerns were minimal. I could change gears.

My husband and I were growing and changing, too. My career focus was shifting. For years, we had worked in close collaboration. At several intervals, we had created innovative enterprises which were highly praised as functional/aesthetic work environments. While these projects were underway, we had spent many hours of the day together at work and at home. Close friends had seen us as "living in each other's pockets." Although our marriage was rich and rewarding much of the time, I needed my own identity. We both did. It was as if we were two seedlings that had been planted in one pot and set out in the sun to grow. Grow we had, far beyond the nurturing capacity of the single pot. It was time to be transplanted into separate pots that would nourish our enlarged root systems. After twenty-three years, the tiny capillary roots were hopelessly intertwined; separating the plants would be a delicate procedure if each one were to live.

Contemplating this shift was terrifying. The root system bled a lot. It hurt.

Jung speaks of this period as a time of "individuation"; Maslow discusses "the movement towards self-actualization"; I was attracted to the idea that growth is an ongoing process and that self-understanding is an essential part of one's creative unfolding. I felt that each of us could realize talents and capacities that might enable us to create a far more harmonious existence for ourselves. Nevertheless, despite the promise of realizing my unknown potential, it was scary to let go of the familiar and take the plunge into uncharted territory.

During the summer months of 1972, I had traveled in Europe on my own. For the first time in twenty years, I had been without family for an extended time. I recall turning around constantly to see where they were. During that summer, I had many symbolic birth dreams. Images of traveling on boats and trains, passing through tunnels, moving out of caves into the light, losing my clothes, finding new shoes.

These symbolic birth dreams were encouraging me to break out of old patterns, to let go of the secure place, to journey into the unknown. How many times all of us choose to cling to the known, the familiar, to the seemingly secure, unwilling to leave our childhood, a bad relationship, an unrewarding job.

Grof inquired about my dreams and fantasies of the past few days. He described psychedelic drugs, and LSD in particular, as "an amplifier or catalyst which would enable me to explore the deeper recesses of my mind." We talked about letting go. Would I be able to let go during the experience? Surrender to the hidden parts of my unconscious? I wasn't certain. It was quite possible that by controlling my feelings, not allowing them to flood through me, I would resist the experience. My husband and I were finding it difficult to allow the needed transformations in our creative but overly dependent partnership to occur; these changes had to happen if the marriage itself was to survive. How to change it and us? Was it desirable or even possible? Was I about to discover the hidden nature of this entity called Leni?

As we talked, I felt increasingly more at ease. Grof was professional, warm, impressively intelligent. He inspired my confidence. Later, during the session, when it seemed as if I were watching a movie inside my head, I was to cast Grof as the great god Thor, his feet planted firmly in the center of the earth.

The next day, with proverbial butterflies in my stomach, I arrived at the center and met Grof at the appointed time. We talked together in the room that I had been shown the day before. It felt familiar—a pleasant room furnished with couches and chairs and attractive paintings. In fact, it might have been a friend's living room. Even though I was still anxious, I felt refreshed by a long night's sleep, and open to the experience that was to begin. I had been observing my dreams during the preceding weeks, noting the feelings that were aroused. I felt cleansed and prepared for a special rite, akin to ceremonies honored in many cultures.

I sat down on the couch, while Grof put on a record out of the group I had selected and then handed me a glass of water containing the drops of LSD. I put on the earphones Grof handed me, stretched out on the couch and listened to the music, waiting, consciously trying to quiet my mind and my nervous stomach. For a fleeting moment, I recalled a psychiatrist friend's remark about LSD at a brunch many years before. Was I indeed playing Russian roulette? Had the flower children felt like this in the '60s as they downed their "acid" on the street? Was I courting insanity, brain damage, death?

The music came through and released me from that anxious train of thought. The sound was calming, contemplative. It was "Music for Zen Meditation," a favorite record of mine. Gradually, it relaxed me. I recalled Grof's description of music as an important unifying and deepening element to the sessions. Thoughts came and went.

Twenty minutes later, I began to feel the effects of the drug. First, there was a period of abstract imagery in which forms appeared and disappeared kaliedoscopically; sometimes they were free form, sometimes geometric. They spiraled, twisted, whirled. I was totally absorbed in the intertwining of three moving strands. I moved into what seemed to be my body and sensed its form, from the molecular to the cellular and skeletal structure. I was both inside and outside; outside observing my bodily processes, inside experiencing them as they occurred.

The spiraling form with which I identified moved into a dim, enveloping, cavernous space. I felt its boundaries. How long I remained in that space I do not know. Clock time no longer had any meaning nor were there any parameters to time or space. Everything was happening in unlimited dimension. My consciousness swelled and completely filled the space I was occupying. I began to move slowly into a long dark tunnel. The walls moved in and out rhythmically, soft moist tissue contracting and expanding in a pulsating motion. At the end of the tunnel was a translucent, cerulean blue light, layered with lavender and sea green, like the clear blue of the most beautiful spring sky. I was suffused with feelings of excitement and pleasure.

Quite abruptly, without warning, everything changed. Unbearable pressure was exerted on my head and body. The pain I experienced was excruciating. Though I was being pushed from behind by some implacable force, no forward movement was possible. Instead, the soft walls closed in. All movement stopped. I was caught in a viselike grip—suffocating—too tiny and powerless a being to fight the unseen force. In an anguished cry, a mixture of rage and fear, I heard myself calling out in the session, "Help me, I'm too small, I can't breathe, I can't make it alone. Why have you abandoned me? Where are you? I need you." For what seemed an unending time, I felt I would die—alone, abandoned, imprisoned in the dark airless cage. There was no exit. I couldn't go forward and I couldn't go back.

Then, as inexplicably as it had stopped, the movement started again. The pulsation was intense and rhythmic. The soft walls moved in and out again . . . opening and closing around me. I actually began to struggle—thrashing about, whimpering and often crying in pain. Grof moved closer, sitting beside me on the couch, stroking my arm gently to reassure me. He didn't speak or intrude. I was simply aware that he was there. As my physical struggle became more intense, he cradled my head against his side. He seemed to sense I wanted something firm to push against; it was quite true. Although I was exerting all my strength, I couldn't push hard enough.

Strains of music wafted through my consciousness. It suited what was happening to me. I didn't try to identify it. Once or twice, I recall, Grof whispered into my ear underneath the headphones, "It's O.K. Don't resist it. Experience it fully, whatever it is." Reassured by his presence, I resumed the titanic battle.

After what seemed like endless time, quite suddenly the struggle ceased and I burst out of my prison into a circle of clear blue light. It was an agonizing expulsion, accompanied by intense pain in my head and neck. I gasped for breath.

I lay still, painfully aware of my breathing. I was free. Exhausted, but free. I moved into a state of euphoria, feeling light and happy. For an undefined period, I was cradled by Grof, wanting nothing more than to be held. At moments, it seemed that I was not breathing at all. Everything was in stasis. I was a totally dependent being. Then I would become frightened and a whole other chain of emotions would begin in me . . . increasing sadness followed by tears, a sense of abandonment and despair . . . then the cycle would begin once again—struggle, pain, the sense of being caged—changing into a feeling of release, euphoria, peace, light. These sensations continued to play themselves out like my own personal movie inside my head, continuing for hours, reels and reels of images appearing until the day was over, unfolding in a series of changing scenes, characters and events. About six o'clock, eight hours after I had taken it, the drug began to wear off. However, the intensified feelings continued. As the rush of images abated, I was more able to take the feeling that had been evoked. The incredible kaleidoscope of memories, of feelings and events remained with me for a long time in quite remarkable detail. The joy, the sadness, the glory and the terror, the present and future were experienced as an incredible array of sequences parading through my mind and emotions. I have returned to it many times to unravel its metaphor and meaning. My perceptions and attitudes shifted, creating a whole new lens through which to view my experience. I realize that my avenue of personal exploration might not be suitable for everyone. However, it was fruitful for me in terms of understanding myself and my life, as well as providing me with insights into the work I ultimately chose to do.

In the first and subsequent sessions with Grof, I discovered within myself a complex inner world, rich in sensibility, symbol, feeling and metaphor not only for those accessible recollections of my childhood and more recent past and those more deeply stored in my unconscious, but also for those that transcended my own direct experience. It was as if the events of my life and the lives of my forebears and unknown people from earlier periods of time and of diverse cultures were passing before me. And even further, I gained an understanding of experience beyond my own physical bodily boundaries, making it apparent that we are all part of a large human family and of an interdependent universal order.

> I became aware that there exists a world of infinite dimension in which I and everything else exists in a complex web of relationship that is interconnected and interpenetrating. That there is, as the new physics teaches us, a basic oneness in the universe. It was this concept that infused the work I was to do.

Later that evening, Grof and I talked about that first session—about the images and events and the feelings they had evoked. It was like opening the floodgates—and was just the beginning of many talks. Mostly, I wanted to sit quietly and contemplate the day's happenings and the emotions that were stirring within me. As I settled into the present, I found myself in a wondrous emo-

tional state . . . everything freshly perceived, senses expanded.
Later, surrounded by close, affectionate companions, the tastes,
smells, textures and visual beauty of dinner were relished. The
world seemed exquisite. Although I went to bed early, it was hours
before I fell asleep. Slowly, the multileveled awareness dimmed.

The next morning, Grof and I met to analyze the session. My
years of psychoanalysis and self-inquiry helped me to work with
the material the session had evoked. In particular, we reviewed
the early part of the morning which I have detailed here.

Could it be that I reexperienced my birth, that I had
symbolically moved through the birth canal and had
been expelled from the womb? Could it possibly be that
so many years after that event, I had brought to a
conscious level the preverbal memory of my birth?

With these questions in mind, I decided to approach my
mother as soon as possible for help in reconstructing the events of
the day of my birth. Amazingly, I had never thought to ask her for
any of these details before—as I'm sure is true for many of us.

In retrospect, it seemed quite remarkable to me that I had so
clearly perceived my mother as my opponent during the LSD
birth experience, involved as we had been in a joint endeavor.
What if there were a grain of truth in my perceptions? Had she
"given up" during labor in the face of overwhelming obstacles? If
so, for what reason had she abandoned me in the middle of the
journey, leaving me to feel as if I had to perform the monumental
task alone?

I was later to discover that she in fact had been literally
abandoned by her maternity nurse. When Grof and I talked,
residual feelings of rage, yearning and frustration flooded me.

As we talked, I tried to connect those feelings with anything I
knew about my birth. I knew little of the actual details, although it
was true that fear of abandonment had indeed motivated a good
deal of the behavior in my life. It was an aspect that had been

dealt with during my Freudian analysis, years earlier. Examining patterns of my behavior was not an unfamiliar process.

I recalled many instances in which it had been necessary to give up a known situation for the unknown. In each case, although I was eager to begin, I became stuck in the middle of the transition, feeling that I was pitted against impossible odds with little trust that I could depend on help from others. Often, minor disappointments were experienced as dramatic instances of abandonment even when I knew my reactions had no logical basis. I went to great lengths to avoid the slightest possibility of being abandoned or left to "go it alone."

It was intriguing that my pervading fear of abandonment might have originated in my birth experience, but this was only speculation without the details that only my mother could provide. So, with the fresh sensory recollection of that "prebirth" and birthing experience, I went to my mother for her factual recollection. We had never discussed my birth before and it was surprising to see how vividly and in what detail she remembered her labor and delivery of so many years ago. I was later to discover that this recall is typical of many women.

My mother recounted the fear and anxiety she had felt in anticipation of my delivery; the birth of my older sister, two years earlier, had been painful and long and she remembered being left for long hours alone in the labor room amidst the groans and screams of other laboring women. The nurses were busy, impersonal, and offered little emotional support. The experience had left her quite frightened. In view of her anxiety, my father had arranged for a private nurse and a private room to support her through the "anguish" of the second birth.

When she arrived at the hospital in the early stages with me, she had been walked up and down the halls according to the practice of the day, until the birth waters broke. She remembered that the doctor came to examine her about ten A.M. and warned the nurse that when the bag of waters broke, the baby would come fast. At about eleven o'clock, lunchtime for the private nurse, Mother was put to bed in her private room, patted on the head as if she were a child and told by her private nurse to hold on tight until she and the doctor returned from their lunch-hour break. Alone and frightened, my mother lay rigid in her narrow hospital bed, tensing every muscle in her body in hopes that she could hold me back until they returned, terrified that I might be born as she lay there alone and unattended in that strange room. When the nurse returned an hour later, bringing the doctor with her, my mother relaxed her hold on me. She was taken to the delivery room. I was born twenty minutes later. "Can you imagine, as a final assault," said my mother, remembering that long past experience, "that the nurse was disgusted that you were a girl and expressed her disappointment quite vocally. When I had trouble nursing you and sought her help, she said not to worry, it didn't matter if I didn't succeed since the baby was *just* a female."

How long do those psychological traces remain with us to govern our responses? Are these reactions imprinted on us and passed onto the generations that follow? Nightmares experienced when we are sleeping prove that we need not be conscious to experience fear and mental anguish. Do we each carry with us frightening, repressed memories of our own births? Indications are that we do. Does it matter? Is it important? I believe that it is. Birth deserves a place on the map of formative events in human consciousness.

Historical Background, Current Theories

Birth *is* the primal event for each of us, and Grof's investigations are not the first attempts to explore these different questions. Psychologists since Freud and Rank—and before that, philosophers and poets from the East and West—have long been telling us that being born is the earliest and most profound emotional shock to our psyches and bodies and may establish response patterns for future transitions that occur during the rest of our lives. Is it an ordeal so profound that its only parallel is death? Many suggest, in fact, that our fear of death begins at birth. Says Grof, "The similarity between birth and death, the startling realization that the beginning of life is the same as its end is the major philosophic issue that accompanies the perinatal [around birth] experience."

Being born is our first and most basic experience; yet, it has been the one to which we have given least attention in our analyses of individual psychological development. Perhaps the techniques now being developed by various therapists will give us the tools to bring our earliest memories to consciousness. It would be valuable for each of us to know about the circumstances of our first nine months in the womb, in order to understand the factors that have made us who we are from the very beginning. Like the ancient Chinese, we might consider that our "birthdays" are marked from the time of conception. From my experience with Grof, it is quite conceivable that we are aware beings in the womb and that our unconscious retains and stores the memory of that period.

Access to these prenatal memories is provided not only through LSD therapy as practiced by Grof, but by many other non-drug therapies such as hypnotic age regression, and body therapies like those pioneered by Wilhelm Reich in the '30s and expanded by Elizabeth Fehr in her combination of hypnosis and body movement rebirthing therapy. Her techniques are being further developed by British psychotherapist R. D. Laing. The "primal therapy" of Janov encourages participants to express or confront the physical pain of the birth shock, utilizing techniques of breathing and vocalizing designed to break through the body armor that, Janov believes, begins to form at birth in reaction to our first—primal—trauma.

Although these methods are still exploratory processes that differ in their approaches, they are all based on the same fundamental idea: birth is one of our primary formative experiences and as such deserves our serious attention.

Consideration of birth as an important aspect of the study of human psychology in the Western world is relatively recent, if one recalls that it was in the 1920s that Sigmund Freud and his disciple, Otto Rank, were debating its importance and its handling in psychoanalysis. Although it was Freud who said, "All anxiety goes back originally to the anxiety of birth," and suggested that the pain of being born and the threat of suffocation during birth was a basic model for later attacks of fear, he did not pursue this aspect of anxiety in his work. However, Rank was deeply influenced by this idea and it became a cornerstone of his philosophy. *The Trauma of Birth* outlines his theory, stressing the traumatic effect of the separation of mother and child, which he called "the primal castration."

Rank emphasized the traumatic aspects of transition from the peace and security of the womb to the harsh realities of extrauterine life. "To be born is to be cast out of the Garden of Eden," said Rank, "and there follows a continuous effort to return to that lost paradise." "The primal anxiety" created by the birth trauma, somehow "blots out the memory of the former pleasurable state." It is the first experience of repression and selective memory. Most of our childhood, claims Rank, is required to overcome the trauma. The primal anxiety which originates at birth is free-floating and may transfer itself to almost any source. As children, we try to discharge the unreleased anxiety by acting it out again and again. Consciously and unconsciously, we seek catharsis or to recapture the security of the womb as we rock in chairs, are carried in planes and boats, float about in lakes and oceans or seek the warm comfort of our baths and beds, in order to effect a cure. Other psychotherapists and researchers through the years have come to share Rank's view of the power of the birth experience to affect later behavior. Forty years later, we are witnessing a renewal of interest in Rank's ideas. New therapies are being devised to help us recognize and work through the effects of the birth trauma.

In the last two decades, important material in support of Rank's point of view has come from contemporary clinical work. Research psychoanalysts such as Grof, and clinical therapists, have repeatedly described the occurrence of birth experiences during patient sessions. Unable to demonstrate literal "memory recall," they usually consider these experiences "allegorical birth fantasies." However, in spite of the otherworldly quality of these experiences, and the prevalence of symbolic and archetypical images, there is often striking agreement with the actual physical aspects of the subject's birth. In addition, details are often substantiated by parental accounts, such as my mother's.

Other examples of birth memories are reported by therapists who employ hypnotic regression, Gestalt therapy, Reichian and bioenergetic body therapies, primal scream therapies and various rebirthing techniques such as the late Elizabeth Fehr's, mentioned earlier. My own "rebirthing" under Fehr's guidance occurred several years after my work with Grof. Fehr, a clinical psychologist, had been recommended to me by friends who knew of my interest in the psychological consequences of birth. Her method had developed from observations of a particularly blocked patient whose body posture in the course of several sessions suggested to her the possibility of a difficult birthing experience. Pursuing that hunch, she guided him through a hypnotic regression over a period of many months, which led him all the way back to birth. This therapy ultimately released him from his nonproductive behavior and provided her with a creative new direction for her own clinical explorations.

She used means quite different from Grof's to release unconscious material—a thirty-foot foam rubber "birth canal" to travel down and a series of directions to guide her patients. Nevertheless, the way I responded physically resembled patterns I had displayed under Grof's observation. As before, I became immobilized near the end of the "birth reenactment," again reflecting what happened during my own birth. However, Fehr's method included continual suggestions that the experience could be reshaped and the old nonproductive memories erased: "It's all right," said Dr. Fehr, sitting beside me, reassuring me.

I believe you had trouble in your birth at this particular

point right before delivery. Do you know that is so? But
this time you can create a new way.

She touched me tenderly. It took all the energy I could muster
and I got myself moving again. I traveled the rest of the way with
the help of my womb companion, another group member acting as
a guide.

Dr. Carl Whitaker, an eminent psychiatrist and family therapist at the University of Wisconsin Medical School, recently said
to me:

> Back in the days when we were using intensive
> regression as a modality of psychotherapy, I went
> through the birth experience with many psychotics and
> many "normal" people. I was always too embarrassed to
> talk about these experiences because I felt that nobody
> except the patient and my colleagues at the clinic would
> believe that these people were really reexperiencing their
> own birth.

A well-known hypnotic researcher and longtime obstetrician,
Dr. David Cheek of San Francisco, has been using age regression
hypnosis for many years as a technique for releasing suppressed
memories of the birth trauma which he feels to be at the root of
many medical symptoms of adult patients. Former president of
the American Society for Clinical Hypnosis, Cheek believes, as do
others, that patients are able to recall and reenact preverbal
experience in trance states.

The concept of "imprinting" is relevant here. As defined by
the noted animal behaviorist Konrad Lorenz, imprinting is the
process by which a young animal transfers its inborn behavior
patterns to an object other than its natural parents. For example,
a young greylag goose reared from the egg by Lorentz responded
to him as if he were its mother, by following him about and in
every respect acting as if Lorenz were its natural parent.

It is Cheek's hypothesis that some kind of imprinting process may occur during the human birth experience, such that in later life we react unconsciously, in negative ways, to stimuli that resemble those present during our birth. Acute claustrophobia, for example, could originate from a difficult birth when strangulation may have been a real possibility. Obviously, some of these "imprinted" behaviors are neither desirable nor useful to us as adults. However, says Cheek, unlike animals, human beings can simulate the recreation of an event, and in the process can envision a more appropriate handling of the experience. In agreement with Fehr, Cheek contends that we may have the ability to alter this so-called "imprinting" and develop new behavior patterns.

The key to this process may lie in our ability to simulate, or reexperience, events such as our own birth. I should emphasize that Grof himself is careful to distinguish between the concepts of intrauterine "memory" and "experience," as in the following excerpt from his book, *Realms of the Human Unconscious.* The important point is that, since it is virtually impossible to verify that a patient is recalling the actual events of his or her birth, the most one can say is that during the LSD session the patient is experiencing the sensation of birth. Whether the therapeutically experienced birth resembles the actual historical birth cannot, of course, be proven. Grof addresses himself directly to this question:

As in the case of the reliving of childhood and birth memories, the authenticity of recaptured intrauterine events is an open question. It seems, therefore, more appropriate to refer to them as experiences rather than memories. I would like to stress, however, that I have tried to be completely open-minded about these phenomena. Whenever it was possible, I have made attempts at objectively verifying such episodes, no matter how absurd these attempts might have appeared to my colleagues. The task was even more difficult than in the case of childhood memories. However, on several occasions, I was able to get surprising confirmations by independently questioning the mother or other persons involved; it should be emphasized that this was done with all the precautions necessary to avoid any contamination of the data. Scientists from various disciplines, such as psychologists and biologists, who volunteered for the LSD training program expressed astonishment at how convincing and authentic these experiences could be. These same sophisticated subjects usually emphasized that experiences of this kind occurred in their sessions in spite of the fact that, before the sessions, they did not accept the possibility of prenatal memories; moreover, the existence of such phenomena was contrary to their presession scientific beliefs.

Stanislav Grof's work with me and other subjects in the '60s and '70s has dramatically augmented our previous knowledge concerning the nature of the "birth trauma." Grof's work has also led scientists, like Carl Sagan in his book *Broca's Brain,* to ask how much, in fact, we do remember of our perinatal experience, and what the consequences of those memories—painful or otherwise—might be:

> We must ask why such recollections are possible—why, if the perinatal experience has produced enormous unhappiness, evolution has not selected out the negative psychological consequences . . . the answer might be that the pros outweigh the cons—perhaps the loss of a universe to which we are perfectly adjusted motivates us powerfully to change the world and improve the human circumstance. Perhaps that striving, questing aspect of the human spirit would be absent if it were not for the horrors of birth.

Grof hypothesizes that there are four basic stages from prenatal life through delivery, which he has called "perinatal matrices." Perinatal (*around birth*) is a word he uses to include the period before, during and immediately after birth. Grof describes the stages that the baby moves through in its relationship to its mother, and that his subjects reexperience metaphorically, as: 1) Primal Union, 2) Antagonism, 3) Synergism and 4) Separation. To arrive at these stages, he has correlated the actual physiological development and events of these periods with the relived experiences of his many subjects.

Grof's thesis has far-reaching significance because he believes that we continue to pass through similar stages as we move through major life transformations. It is parallel to the major theory of anthropologist Arnold Van Gennup, which in the early 1900s formulated (from an anthropological point of view) stages of adult transition—rites of passage such as: puberty, marriage, childbirth, retirement, old age and dying.

In addition, we are discovering that individual rites of passage, such as mourning the deaths of people close to us, have their own distinct reponse patterns, as shown by Kübler-Ross's pioneering work. An understanding of these patterns can give us structure and comfort as we cope with the impact of what would otherwise be almost impossible to accept. Traditional rituals, customs and ceremonies at these crucial times, in more stable cultures, have always provided this support. Grof's ideas include, yet go beyond, these earlier views of behavior during transitional periods.

In the *Primal Union* stage described by Grof, the child floats in its mother's ocean protected by the uterine sac, its needs provided for through the umbilical cord, moving in symbiotic harmony with its mother. A feeling of oceanic ecstasy pervades. Its mother's activities can affect this tranquil environment, however. If the mother overeats, drinks alcohol, or smokes, for example, she can profoundly disturb this otherwise protected inner universe. Disturbances that we normally consider only as a source of physiological stress may also be experienced on a primitive psychological level as well. And, if assaults are continual, they create the impression of a "bad womb." When subjects relive periods of intrauterine disturbance, they often report headaches, chills and nausea that may have been part of the original experience.

Grof's subjects also describe a variety of normal uterine sensations: they feel extremely small, and are aware of the disproportion between head and body size, the amniotic fluid and the umbilical cord floating after them.

The second stage, _Antagonism with the Mother_, is marked by the onset of uterine contractions. The walls of the uterus begin to contract but the cervix is not yet open. The mother and baby are a source of pain to each other. The unborn child is compressed at intervals for what seems unending time. There appears to be "no exit," no way out in time or space. Many experience this stage as a sensation of being sucked into a cosmic maelstrom or a whirlpool. This memory is then projected onto all life situations in which overwhelming circumstances impose themselves on a seemingly helpless, passive victim.

In the third stage, referred to as _Synergism,_ the efforts of the mother and child again coincide. It is the second clinical stage of labor. The cervix has opened. Yet, as the birth journey unfolds, the baby is subject to intense, crushing pressure and to periods of suffocation as contractions propel it through the birth canal. During this third stage, subjects show physical manifestations strikingly similar to those experienced during actual birth: enormous pressure on head and body, choking, pain in various parts of the body, palpitating heart and complex twisting movements. An end to the agony is near and the mother and child jointly strive to end this mutually painful stage. Intense energy is channeled through the body, and is finally released explosively as the baby's head emerges. The tension seems beyond endurance and transmits into "wild, ecstatic raptures." This becomes a volcanic ecstasy that contrasts with the "oceanic ecstasy" of the first stage.

The fourth stage—_Separation from the Mother_—is related to the moment of birth. The ordeal of the journey is over, the first breath is taken, the umbilical cord is cut, the infant begins life as an autonomous being. There is sudden relief and relaxation. People often relive this stage of the birth in amazing sensory detail, including smells of hospital rooms and anesthesia, metallic sounds of surgical instruments, even conversations, and the brightness of the lighting.

49

The general acceptance of religious ideas, it seems to me [speculates Carl Sagan in Broca's Brain], *can only be because something in them resonates with our own certain knowledge—something deep and wistful; something every person recognizes as central to our being. And that common thread, I propose, is birth. Religion is fundamentally mystical, the gods inscrutable, the tenets appealing but unsound because, I suggest, blurred perceptions and vague premonitions are the best that the newborn infant can manage. . . . All successful religions seem at their nucleus to make an unstated and perhaps even unconscious resonance with the perinatal experience.*

The death-rebirth struggle is the most significant aspect of this final period and represents the termination and resolution of the birth process. The entire world seems to be collapsing; all reference points disappear. Eastern philosophy refers to this as "ego death"—total annihilation of the individual on all imaginable levels—physical, emotional, intellectual, moral and transcendental. The ego death is followed by visions of white or golden light and feelings of enormous decompression and expansion. The subject feels cleansed and purged, freed from anxiety and aggressive impulses. Enhanced self-esteem is accompanied by appreciation for others, a sense of love and a general affirmation of existence. If the quality of mothering in these first postnatal moments is high, this final stage comes full circle and can approximate the first stage of bliss. Similarly, as in Fehr's method, a nurturing therapist can intercede at this point in the adult's rebirthing to provide the positive mothering that can help the subject complete the process and therefore move beyond it.

Other clinical research corroborates Grof's findings. Dr. Frank Lake, an English psychoanalyst who works with LSD, observes similar patterns of recall.

In the early stages of labor, Lake observes, the unborn child is strongly motivated toward birth and perseveres in the arduous process, but as the passage becomes more and more difficult, there is an equally strong desire to return to familiar life in the womb. During the second stage, going forward and going backward seem equally impossible, and it is then that an innate will to live, a life force, appears to take over. It is an existential crisis.

In the 1940s psychoanalyst Nandor Fodor offered some of the insights that have led to the development of present thinking about birth trauma. Far ahead of his time, Fodor offered some basic principles concerning birth trauma in his book, *Search for the Beloved*:

1. Birth is now almost always traumatic.
2. The longer labor takes and the more serious the physical complications, the greater the trauma of birth.
3. The intensity of the trauma of birth is proportionate to the shocks or injuries which the child suffers during labor or immediately following delivery.
4. The love and care which the child receives immediately after birth is a decisive factor in the persistence and intensity of traumatic stress.

In the 1970s French obstetrician Frederick Leboyer came to similar conclusions. Some years earlier while undergoing analysis, after twenty years of traditional obstetrical practice in Paris, Leboyer became painfully aware of the traumatic effects of his own birth. The development of his ideas and his now well-known method (which he adamantly explains is not a method, but an attitude—a protocol for birth) emerged out of the reexperiences of his own thirty-hour biological labor in which he "felt" he was facing death. As a result of psychoanalysis and his study of Buddhism in India and Europe, he became more psychologically aware, identifying subsequently with the baby's titanic struggle into life. Out of this awareness have come three books and a film which describe his "nonviolent" approach to birth.

Some suggest, in agreement with Fodor and Leboyer and others, that postnatal physical contact is so integral a part of the birth process that it may be seen as the fourth stage of labor and should be considered as part of the delivery process.

These ideas again bring up the question of our own psychological "imprinting" just after birth. That the period after birth is a highly significant one for the emotional well-being of the baby has been shown by the pioneering work of Marshall Klaus and John Kennell at Case Western Reserve Medical School in Cleveland. Their films of mother-child interaction clearly demonstrate the instinctive "getting acquainted" process, the repetitive ritualistic pattern that we now refer to as "bonding." Intriguingly, most new mothers follow the same sequence in handling and caressing their nude babies. As the mother strokes and fondles her baby against her own body, she welcomes it into the world. She examines it minutely and identifies it, exploring by touch the baby she has carried for nine months, discovering on the outside the person she has known inside her body.

Klaus believes that as the mother touches her baby, gazes into its eyes, soothes its naked body, so sensitized from the trauma of its birth, she is going through a ritual of "knowing" it to be hers. The Sufis say one must avert one's gaze from the eyes of the newborn until the baby has looked into the eyes of the mother; otherwise, it is an interference in the natural order of life.

Klaus and Kennell found that women who were able to have such early extended physical contact with their babies formed deeper attachments than mothers who were not permitted, because of hospital regulations, to perform this bonding ritual. This "bonding" period has been well documented for animals by scientists like Lorenz who discovered that brief periods of partial or complete separation after birth may drastically distort a mother animal's feeding and caring for her infant. The work of Klaus and Kennell, among others, has forced a thorough review of perinatal practices and caused many American hospitals to alter their former routines. The trauma of birth *is* lessening in this and other ways.

My work with Grof affected me profoundly, as did his book *Realms of the Human Unconscious*. My perceptions and attitudes shifted dramatically. I began to perceive new connections between events in my life and saw my own experiences as continuous and interrelated rather than mysterious and random. My sense of personal order expanded to include a deeper awareness of the miraculous order and patterns in the external world. Not only did I become more connected to my own self but that self became more connected to everything beyond. The concepts of harmony and continuity became guiding themes for me. It was through this personal journey that I came to be so intensely interested in the circumstances surrounding pregnancy—the environment of birth and the pregnant year. Although I realized that my particular avenue of exploration might not be the choice of many others, it was appropriate for me at that time in my life.

I came to understand that "birth" is not a single event but a process which begins at conception, is established at implantation and embraces nine months in the womb. The final stage—which we now call birth—is the momentous journey down the birth canal toward a separate existence. In those first nine months, I believe, we experience the sense of oneness—the oceanic bliss—at the same time that we suffer the opposite sensations: earthbound discomforts caused by our mother's activities as she copes with the complex demands of her daily life. This is our first intimation of the balance of opposites that exist in the world we will enter.

The birth process, viewed in this way, became for me a demonstration of how the world works, presenting us with a metaphor, a map—the symbol standing for the whole. Before we know, we "know."

As a result of my session with Grof, which connected me to my own birth, the focus of my Ph.D. study changed. I moved my attention to the earliest period of our existence when we are subject to influences that forever affect our lives. It was stunning to contemplate how this realization could alter the ways in which we as individuals and as a culture might choose to shape our experience of pregnancy and birth.

I found myself wanting to know more about the developmental changes that occur during pregnancy. Before we can even contemplate ways to design a more nurturing environment for this transformational period, we must try to understand the biological, psychological and spiritual dimensions of this rite of passage. The next two chapters present some new ideas about the developmental changes of the childbearing year, first, from the point of view of the baby, and then from the parents' perspective.

II

Nine Months of Change: The Person Developing in the Womb

There is no particular moment when life begins, there is only gradual elaboration of the potentialities ultimately inherent in every cell . . . there is no physiological infusion of life at a given point . . . there is only growth.

Joshua Lederberg,
Nobel Laureate

One mother says her baby was born patient, serene, a contemplative little philosopher. A father says his daughter was a squirming, restless acrobat from the first moment.

It's clear—newborn babies differ in a variety of observable ways. Because there have been no experiences outside the womb to exert their influence, these differences can be traced to the combined effects of three factors: the basic genetic endowment bestowed by the parents, the normal course of an individual's intrauterine development, and the circumstances of birth itself. But what *are* the possible influences on development in the womb? We know the "preborn child" and its maternal environment begin interacting at conception in a process that continues throughout adult life:

Slowly, the old nature-nurture controversy—the question as to whether heredity or environment is more important—is being recognized as a nonissue. What is emerging instead is a complementary theory of life, where genes and environment work together. The genes determine the range of potential possibilities: and the environment selects among them. Thus, for example, genes may dictate that someone grows to a height between five-feet-eight-

57

inches and six-feet-one-inch; but diet, hygiene, stress and general health will determine the precise point at which growth stops.

Dr. Zsolt Harsanyi, Cornell Medical Center, and Richard Hutton, medical writer

Although the myriad factors that create the known differences between infants at birth have yet to be—and may never be—completely clarified, the brain and nervous system of the baby is the basis of the baby's future awareness of its surroundings. All the incredible human faculties that help us make sense of the world—speech, sensory perceptions, memory, self-awareness—depend on complicated interactions within our nervous system.

How does this core of awareness develop? Surely, not all at once at the moment of birth? Does the unborn child have self-awareness? We may not yet know the answers to these difficult questions, but we know enough, as this chapter will relate, to cause us to seriously reevaluate our current thinking about the nature of the unborn child.

Is the quality of life in the womb one of the influences on our later behavior?

Although the fundamental question of fetal consciousness and how its development is influenced has been explored and expounded upon for centuries by philosophers, poets and mystics, it is a question medical science has largely ignored. In 1968, the eminent biochemist Rene Dubos expressed his concern over this state of affairs in an interview published in the *Journal of the American Medical Association*. He emphasized that until very recently it was customary to regard fetal and neonatal states as relatively unaffected by the external environment, except for instances where infection or other obvious threats existed. However, Dubos stressed, we now know that subtle variations in the biological environment, factors relevant to the environment of the mother, can profoundly affect growth, development and even the personality of the child.

This viewpoint is being accepted, albeit slowly. Most practicing physicians—and, more to the point, most obstetricians—learn little during their early training concerning prenatal awareness. Medical texts still deal primarily with pathology, abnormality and disease. Roger Stevenson, author of a standard text on the fetus and the newborn, explained the situation in 1973 in the preface of his book, *The Fetus and Newly Born Infant*.

Indeed, the earliest recognized environmental influence, that of psychologic experiences of the mother, has not been discussed (here). This results from the paucity of controlled data on the subject rather than its lack of importance.

Meanwhile, as speculation continues, a body of scientific data is finally beginning to accumulate to help us map the baby's prenatal experience, trimester by trimester. There are signs of a new focus of attention in the founding of the journal *Early Human Development* in the late 1970s. The editors describe it as an international journal "concerned with the continuity of fetal and postnatal life." A quote resurrected from a 1902 Scottish antenatal pathology manual affirms the journal's viewpoint: "Truly, birth marks not a beginning but a stage in life's journey." (J. W. Ballantyne, 1902)

Although it is apparent that for quite a long time poets, mystics and some scholars have recognized the importance of the prenatal period, it is only recently that medical science has begun to systematically study the mystery of our beginnings, following its time-honored studies of the life cycles of other species and its inquiries into many other aspects of human biology and experience. A new term, psychoembryology, gives status to the field (within the larger discipline of fetology) which seeks to analyze human psychological development from conception on.

The invention of the microscope in the seventeenth century enabled us to observe living organisms in more minute detail than was previously possible and to unravel, via the microscope, some of life's mysteries. More recently, medical researchers like Lennart Nilsson, Swedish pioneer of scientific medical photography and author of A Child Is Born, and Dr. Motoyuki Hayashi, head of Obstetrics and Gynecology at Tokyo's Toho University School of Medicine, have developed ways of filming its biological inception, using advanced instruments, time-lapse photography and hysterscope (a tool that permits observation of hollow organs, in this case, the womb) and filming pregnant rabbits and monkeys.

A concrete side effect of this basic research is that women who want a full-term, normal pregnancy may benefit if their doctors are able to apply useful information gleaned during such studies. Much of what has been learned in fetology also comes from the study of pregnant mice and rabbits.

Medical researchers, such as New Zealand obstetricians Doctors H. M. I. Liley and A. William Liley, a husband and wife team, have contributed to our knowledge through their observations in their research with unborn babies suffering from the acute anemia caused by mother-child blood (Rh factor) incompatibility. Other important data has been gathered through diagnostic and treatment techniques developed to detect and solve life-threatening fetal disorders. Amniocentesis, which is removal of ten to twenty milliliters of amniotic fluid by means of a hollow needle inserted into a pregnant woman's uterus, is the most common form of prenatal diagnosis. Immediate testing of the fluid, or culturing of cells in the fluid, can reveal the presence of genetic syndromes such as sickle cell anemia or Down's syndrome. Also, ultrasound (sonarography) is sometimes used to reveal structural abnormalities or patterns of movement. These exploratory techniques developed through medical research are also being used to learn more about the biology and sensory responses of the child in the womb.

It is surprising to realize, in fact, that obstetrics, pediatrics and gynecology, those specialized branches of medicine that care for women and children are only about sixty years old and that the field of fetology, devoted to the care and understanding of the baby from conception to birth, is only about fifteen years old.

Of course, there have been serious studies made of fetal behavior for many years, even before the discipline had a name. Early researchers in this field include L. W. Sontag and others at the Fels Research Institute in Yellow Springs, Ohio. Sontag suggests that one reason little consideration has been given to behavior in the womb and the environmental factors that influence it may be our difficulty in accepting the idea that "the human psyche might know of its own coming."

Yet Eastern thought, with its belief in reincarnation, has accepted the idea of womb consciousness for centuries. In a Tibetan text from about 1100 A.D., there is a detailed description that begins with the earliest stages of consciousness as the ovum and sperm meet and the embryo forms. It delineates the feelings of the unborn human person as it develops week by week—a description of pain and agony, in contrast to the theory of womb life as oceanic bliss accepted in Western thought.

Each society evolves a particular view about the genesis of life and of death that harmonizes with its total philosophy and organization, which then determines cultural attitudes and myths and behavior in relation to childbearing. The philosophy and the behavioral patterns become woven together, creating the society which then influences the next generation. Each society thus has characteristic effects on the environment of the womb from the earliest moments of development. What is crucial is that we begin to see that growth and development are continuous processes. Conception is only the beginning of a cycle that continues our whole lives.

Even standard textbooks for medical students are beginning to view life as a continuum:

Development is a continuous process that begins when an ovum is fertilized by a sperm and ends at death. It is a process of growth and differentiation which transforms a single cell into a multicellular adult human being. Most developmental changes occur during the embryonic and fetal period, but important changes also occur during infancy, childhood, adolescence and adulthood.

Although it is customary to divide development into *prenatal* and *postnatal* periods, it is important to realize that birth is merely a dramatic event during development resulting in a distinct change in environment. Development does not stop at birth.

Keith L. Moore,
The Developing Human

In this chapter we will look at the development of the baby in the womb in terms of its progressively more complicated behavior patterns. Then we will examine some of the evidence that psychological development in the womb may be more subject to external environmental factors than has commonly been believed until recently. In a sense, we are witnessing a resurgence in the old belief of the power of "maternal impressions" to affect the baby's development, although we now think in terms of mediating influences such as the existence of stress-induced hormones to explain what was previously inexplicable.

The conception of a new human being, though an ordinary occurrence, is an extraordinary miracle. The complex process of human development begins with the simple fertilization of the human egg—the fusion of the sperm and the egg. As we know, this fertilized egg contains all the genetic information necessary to produce the adult human being. Within this tiny single-celled human organism, which can only be seen through a magnifying lens, are the genes that we inherit from both our parents. As emphasized earlier, this genetic heritage may determine certain of our characteristics, such as the color of our eyes or blood type, but in many respects it simply provides for a range of possibilities which the environment will shape in ways we do not yet fully understand. For instance, our height will also be affected by our mother's diet during pregnancy, and by our own diet after birth. Attributes such as intelligence and "temperament" are more difficult to analyze, but there is increasing evidence that both heredity and environment play substantial roles.

The most recent research indicates that even the infant in the womb is aware of, and affected by, its immediate environment to a much larger extent than we had believed possible. The question that then arises is: how *soon* does the developing organism become sensitive to its total environment, and what kinds of interactions occur, and how lasting are the effects? Let us look more closely at some stages of fetal development as they are currently understood.

Cell division is initiated by fertilization, and the genetic information then begins to express itself, following genetically programmed signals that we do not yet fully understand. For example, at the twelve or sixteen cell stage, called the morula, the cells all appear to be identical, but will give rise to very different tissues. The outer layer of the morula will develop into the placenta, and the inner layer will form the basis of the embryo itself. The elementary foundation of the central nervous system does not begin to form until after the second week of development, but once begun, change is rapid.

The central theme throughout the development of the baby's central nervous system and other body organ structures is that there is a strict time sequence involved. Thus, any interference in this developmental process will have extremely different results depending on the point when the interference occurs. Influences are potentially positive or negative.

There is copious medical documentation of development that goes wrong because of either faulty genes or diseases contracted during pregnancy, such as rubella. Similarly, pregnant women can now benefit from extensive published research on the deleterious effects of radiation, drugs, alcohol, smoking and poor nutrition on fetal development. Much less well understood are the possible effects of more subtle environmental factors such as stress, noise, lights, etc. on human development—or of meditation, biofeedback, or simply maintaining a calm, tranquil environment during pregnancy.

Much is known about the development of the physical body structures of the baby in the womb—but what is known of the development of the earliest human behavior? Clearly, we need to know what makes up the normal range of behavioral changes in order to begin to understand how external factors may impinge on and change behavior patterns.

Behavior Patterns in the Womb

Donald H. Barron, who worked in Cambridge, England, and at Yale University during the 1940s, described three distinct stages of mammalian development which he calls the *inactive, active* and *reactive* stages. During the first, *inactive stage*, no movement occurs at all. Then, when the skeletal muscles have become responsive to direct electrical stimulation, the organism is able to respond with movement.

The next stage is called the *active stage* because there is more spontaneous activity, which is very similar in pattern among a variety of mammalian species. It is possible that these seemingly spontaneous movements are really primitive reactions to external stimuli. However, at this point in development, reflex pathways have not been established. Movements in this stage tend to be characterized by slow bending of the neck and trunk.

During the next or *reactive stage*, direct sensory stimulation evokes responses in the muscular system, and reflexes of different types appear. The first reflex can be elicited between the middle of the seventh and the beginning of the eighth week of gestation, Davenport Hooker, an anatomist at the University of Pittsburgh, discovered in his studies.

Between the eleventh and twelfth weeks, the face will move away from a stimulus, instead of merely moving from side to side.

Oral reflexes develop rapidly, from mouth opening at nine and one half weeks to the demonstrated swallowing of amniotic fluid as early as the twelfth week.

At the end of the first trimester, the baby in the womb is three and one half inches long, and weighs one ounce. Its body is active. It is able to kick, twist its feet and even curl its newly emergent toes. Its tiny arms are able to bend at the wrist and at the elbow and its tiny hands can make a fist. Even its face is mobile and it can frown, purse its lips, open its mouth and even squint, despite the fact that the eyes are sealed shut.

At the end of twelve weeks, says Hooker in his book *The Origin of Overt Behavior*, the quality of response is altered; it is an important age landmark. Movements become graceful and fluid as they are in the newborn. Reflexes become more vigorous.

At this point, each baby's behavior is demonstrably individual since the actual structure of muscles, which follows an inherited pattern, varies from baby to baby.

The unborn child sucks its fingers from about fourteen weeks on, and sips the amniotic fluid in which it floats. An analysis of the amniotic fluid shows that it contains protein and sugar. By the eighth and ninth month, if active in the womb, the baby will drink six to eight pints of fluid a day. At the first feeding after birth, the newborn is more practiced than anyone gives it credit for, since it has known for several months how to find its mouth with its fingers. The experience of sucking and swallowing in the womb helps the baby to nurse immediately after birth.

Gradually, the early simple reflexes combine to yield increasingly complex "reactive" patterns until smooth, coordinated behavior emerges.

Beyond the age of twenty-eight weeks, premature infants can survive on their own, and have provided researchers with a basis for describing behavior from this age on. According to Arnold Gesell, Director of the Clinic of Child Development at the Yale School of Medicine, fundamental rates and patterns of development are not altered by birth itself, so it is valid to assume that the behavior of the premature infants parallels that of babies in the womb.

At twenty-eight to thirty-two weeks, Gesell observed that fetal movements are fleeting, with mild avoidance responses to light and sound. There is no definite sleeping or waking pattern.

By thirty-two to thirty-six weeks, there are strong responses to light and sound and periods of definite wakefulness. The emergence of a true sleep-waking cycle in the eighth month is considered by fetologists to be a critically important developmental transition. This is the onset of an adult sleep-waking pattern, which is essential to the healthy function of life as a human and is still not understood.

It is apparent that most of what we know about "behavior" in the womb is based on movement patterns of the unborn baby. Similarly, when we try to analyze how the external environment is affecting the unborn baby, we talk in terms of increased fetal mobility or cardiac rate. For example, if the mother's abdominal wall is stimulated by vibration, the baby in the womb responds with increased movements. As you will see in the next section, some researchers believe that not only sound vibrations, but a mother's fatigue and emotions also affect the unborn child. The unanswerable question that remains, of course, is how the perturbations of normal life felt in the womb ultimately affect the growing fetus, as well as adult response patterns in later life. We do not have the answers yet—but at least we now believe that the question is of vital importance. Just as the experience of a particular smell often sweeps us back to seemingly forgotten incidents or locales, perhaps all our other senses are connected to stored intrauterine sensory experiences, which may be evoked and unconsciously influence our behavior in subtle ways.

Fetology has made great strides since 1963, when a respected book for expectant mothers adamantly asserted that "nothing you think, see or hear during pregnancy will affect your child in the slightest."

We will never know exactly what is experienced in the womb; we may come closest to it through the intuition of poets and philosophers or through insights of the mystics. The poet Samuel Coleridge (and Descartes before him) believed there were probably more experiences of interest and of moment in the first nine months of life than in all the years *after* birth.

Developmental Influences: The Maternal Environment and Beyond

Although it was previously considered that gestation ran through a simple predetermined course of growth and development, we now realize that child and mother influence *each other*, both biologically and emotionally.

The New Zealand researcher-fetologist-physician, Dr. H. M. I. Liley, believes that the fetus is "in command of the pregnancy and is not a passive passenger." She says it is the unborn baby who determines or establishes the endocrine balance during gestation and initiates the necessary physiological changes in the mother's body that ensure a hospitable environment for the new being during the course of pregnancy—the baby assumes which way it will lie in the womb in response to different stimuli; it influences its own birthing time (by individual response to the levels of various hormones passing between it and its mother) and which way it will present in labor. It is said if one observes the position that babies seek as newborns as they lie naked on the bed before falling asleep, one will see their "lie," the position they preferred in the womb.

Within the protective custody of its mother's body, the growing human is learning how to be in the world even as it passes through its rapid stages from embryo to fetus to baby. It experiences the outer environment and even the nature of its culture through its mother's daily interactions in it, and also through its own interactions with the outside world (through the vibrations of the sounds of TV or planes or the cacaphony of conversation). The organism is sophisticated enough to manage incoming information from the environment by responding primitively.

Many of its mother's normal habits and attitudes must be reexamined during pregnancy to insure its oxygen supply and to protect the unborn child. If its mother is a drinker or a smoker, it is adversely affected. Her cigarette habit constricts her blood vessels and reduces the amount of oxygen the baby receives. It might even be born prematurely as a result.

Investigations by Sontag's group in 1935 demonstrated that eight to ten minutes after a mother finishes her cigarette, the fetal heartbeat increases thirty-nine beats per minute. But, more surprising, Dr. Michael Lieberman, in a modification of the Sontag study reported in a 1970 review of prenatal development, demonstrated that even before the mother lit her cigarette and started to smoke, the baby's heartbeat increased in anticipation of the event, simply as a result of the mother being shown the cigarette and reacting to the *idea* of smoking! It is believed that the mother's heartbeat might increase in anticipation to the actual smoking of the cigarette, or that an "adrenal-like drug" might cross the placental barrier and stimulate the fetal heart. At any rate, a definite response occurs. The implications of this observation of an indirect cause-and-effect fetal response are startling and far-ranging.

All kinds of drugs present a problem in the womb. Even aspirin can pass through the mother's bloodstream and filter through to the unborn baby.

Chemical substances in the medication and drugs administered to the mother cross the placental barrier and lodge in the baby's brain and body in very different proportions to the mother's larger structure. The concentration of medication required for the mother's body exceeds the concentration for the child. Her more complex system also has the capacity to break down the drugs she has ingested and to transform them into other substances that can be absorbed into tissues in a useful form. However, babies in the womb do not have this capability. The drugs that pass through to them are not metabolized and affect the babies in quite a different way.

From what we now know, it seems clear that during pregnancy all drugs should be carefully considered and not used unless necessary for the mother's health. In the normal course of our day, we take pills for so many ailments that most of us are unaware of the quantity and variety that we use. Among them are antacids, antihistamines and barbituates. In varying amounts, and at various times during gestation and birth, each of these has been found to have deleterious effects on the development of a baby. New research continually produces additional warnings about the deleterious effects on the mother as well.

Environmental pollution is another hazard to the unborn— the greater the pollution, the less oxygen will pass to the baby through the mother's blood. Gasoline engine exhaust, emissions from factories, chemical plants, airports, pesticides—all are assaults to development and eventually will affect human evolution. The baby receives less oxygen and more harmful pollutants.

The baby is also affected by its mother's temperament and her daily habits as she lives through each day. She receives stimulation from her environment, she reacts, the unborn child receives the stimulation through her body. The womb environment is affected. It is a form of "learning" which changes the baby. Her moods affect the baby who responds differently when she is rushed or relaxed, tense or calm, happy or enraged. The baby's activity shows a marked increase when the mother is emotionally disturbed and is usually quiet when she is at ease. How differentiated these mood tones are, as experienced by the baby, is still open to investigation.

At the Fels Research Institute in Yellow Springs, Ohio, Sontag and his associates discovered, for example, that distress in the mother produces a marked increase in fetal activity. Fatigue does the same.

Severe emotional stress, especially during the later months of pregnancy, tends to produce an exceptionally active, squirming, irritable baby who will have feeding problems. The implications are clear: anything that can be done to ease the stress on the mother will benefit the baby.

The baby hears a great deal of sound in the womb, since auditory capacities develop early. At five months, the auditory nerves carry messages from the ear to the brain. The womb, in fact, is quite a noisy place. The amniotic fluid serves as a more effective sound conductor than air, amplifying the sounds both inside and outside the womb. There is great activity inside the mother's body. The unborn child hears and feels the pulsations of her blood coursing through the arteries and the placenta. It hears the rhythmic pounding of her heart and of its own, which beats twice as fast as hers. And it hears the rumblings of its mother's last meal traveling through her intestines and bowels. We have discovered this through recordings made of sounds inside the body.

Tests have proven that the baby is sensitive to sound at twenty-eight weeks, and its reactions are numerous. It responds actively to various sounds and vibrations. To the baby in the womb, the many sounds together might sound like a fugue. The vibration from a washing machine, for example, can stimulate extreme activity. So also will its mother's tapping vibration on the side of the bathtub as she bathes, or the sound of her typewriter or concert music. In fact, as a result, its heartbeat can increase by ten or more beats per second in response to sounds. Imagine all the other sounds and vibrations we respond to!

Bombarded by sounds in the womb, the baby may begin to select and exercise preferences about what feels comfortable to its "sensibilities." Pregnant women have been forced to leave concerts where too much percussion was played. The babies kicked violently. Dr. T. Berry Brazelton, Associate Professor of Pediatrics at Harvard, observes that when newborn, we exhibit strong preferences immediately after delivery. It is possible that we are simply exhibiting the selective behavior we exercised in our uterine life. For instance, says Brazelton, in the delivery room newborn infants may react to a loud noise once, but, on hearing it the second and third times, will tune it out. It seems babies quickly temper their startle reaction and turn toward a more comfortable sound, such as a soft voice.

Sounds from outside the womb, which comprise a mother's daily activity, affect the unborn every moment. Therefore, prenatal experience may well be patterned in part by mundane things like motion picture sounds, the sound and vibrations of television, voices in family arguments, as well as sonic booms, roaring airplanes and the complex hubbub of the city. Not only do babies hear them directly from the source through the walls of the mother's body and react to their experience of them, but they also receive a double impact of the mother's emotional and physical reaction to them.

In tests performed by Sontag, a startle response was produced in the fetus when a sound was applied to the abdominal wall of the mother. An immediate acceleration of the baby's heart rate accompanied the sound. They concluded that the baby perceived the sound directly rather than the reaction being a result of the mother's perception of the sound, for the change of endocrine products in her blood could not be so rapidly transferred to the baby.

Dr. Henry Truby says that babies overhear their mother's conversations from within the womb. Truby suggests that the linguistic environment of the last few months influences infant speech and language in childhood. Truby, Professor of Pediatrics, Linguistics and Anthropology at the University of Miami, maintains that infants in the womb overhear their mother's conversations. In research done on a sabbatical leave, in Sweden, Truby and his colleagues determined that the fetus hears during the entire last half of its nine months in the womb, perhaps even earlier than the last half. Truby says we carry over "the mother tongue" we heard *in utero* in a subtle accent of speech when we begin to talk. A sound analysis instrument can detect it when it is too subtle for the naked ear. To Truby, this suggests the possibility that some kind of prenatal language learning occurs. From the Institute for Child Development of Stanford University, pediatrician Tom Forrest reports that sonargraphic studies of the fetus show that it moves in synchrony with its mother's voice. These studies both indicate that some patterning of infant behavior may begin even before birth.

We see that before birth babies respond to biochemical influences *and* to environmental ones such as movement, light and sound. They are delicately tuned organisms long before their transition to the outside world.

If the fetus can respond, and, in addition, is in a state of development so that each response is more aptly called learning, then indeed the fetus—in the broadest sense of the word—is learning prior to birth. This must be said cautiously, since we do not learn *in utero* in terms of $1 + 1 = 2$, or ABC, and we do not dream in words. But perhaps marked environmental changes can shape later learning, ability, development and function of the fetal brain.

Mortimer G. Rosen, M.D. and Lynn Rosen, Ed.D., *Your Baby's Brain Before Birth*

For example, researchers trying to explain the preference of human newborns for specifically patterned visual stimuli have come up with a startling hypothesis: prior visual experience with these patterns during intrauterine life determines later adult patterns. Patterns preferred by newborns fall into groups resembling adult "phosphenes," those visual images, characteristic for each person, induced by mechanical or electrical stimulation of the visual system, such as pressing hard on your eyeballs. Anderson, of the University of Nebraska Medical Center, sums up the significance of this idea by pointing out that the characteristic phosphene patterns that an individual sees may be produced by pressure on the visual system; the amount of pressure required varies with age. Therefore, he goes on to suggest, it may be that fetal phosphene patterns are determined by the pressure conditions that exist in the womb; this might explain how a newborn could display preferences for certain combinations of vertical or horizontal lines that are influenced by its experience prior to "birth."

Of interest here is the fact that every time the mother breathes she is varying the intrauterine pressure on her child! Clearly, her emotional state will influence her breathing pattern, so this is a simple example of possible maternal influences on normal development.

In what other ways might the mother's behavior and attitudes affect the unborn child? Does "learning" occur? If so, then can we create conditions in which we can foster feelings of trust, security and love in our children even *before* they are born? It's worth trying.

The possibility that human awareness may begin at conception has profound implications—social, psychological and spiritual ones. The earlier we begin to honor and nurture the developing capacities of this being during its sojourn in the womb, the more likely the baby is to reach its fullest potential as it continues to develop throughout its extrauterine life. As our perceptions of the nature of pregnancy and birth change, so will our behavior and attitudes during the childbearing year. The potential benefits to the developing person are vast. The limits are unknown.

Pregnancy is an incredibly dynamic period. The developing person in the womb is integrally linked to you and to the complex and unique texture of your life. During this transitional state, you are integrally connected to the mystery and miracle of the life process.

Giving birth can be a deeply intimate experience for both partners; it can be a window to intrinsic patterns of the universe, to the cycles of life and death that have existed since the first matter crossed that indefinable boundary line and took the form of living cells.

As parents you can benefit enormously by fostering a harmonious relationship with your baby, your partner and your world during this unique time.

III

One Becomes Two Becomes Three:
Women and Men
Become Mothers and Fathers

In her pregnant state, as a woman becomes a mother, she may feel many things—

- The whole meaning of my life has changed; things will never be the same.
- I feel so sexy, does everybody know?
- I'm afraid I will be this way forever: needy, dependent, emotional, anxious.
- I *want* to be this way forever: peaceful, serene.
- I love being pregnant, but I'm afraid of the responsibility of the child.
- I'll be fat and ugly forever.
- He won't love me anymore; he'll find someone else to love.
- Having a baby will ruin my career.
- I don't know who I am any more.
- I feel slow and stupid.
- I'm an integral part of the universe. It's hard to explain.
- I want a lot of cuddling. I feel like a kitten who wants to be stroked.
- We'll never have any time together after the baby is born.
- I'm afraid I'm going to die.
- It's the first time I've had a purpose in my life.
- Even when *I'm* not doing anything, my body is making a new person!

* * *

Is birth an event or a process? We tend to focus on the actual birth because it is dramatic and because we can see it happening. But, just as for the baby the birth event may be considered a link between two states of consciousness—for the mother, too, it is in reality a bridge between two worlds.

During this period of gestation, while the baby in the womb is making its remarkable journey into becoming, a mother is also undergoing an extraordinary process directly related to the child's growth within her. A body of knowledge is accumulating that helps us map the complex dimensions of her altered state during the childbearing year. We are becoming increasingly aware that childbearing can precipitate transcendent, ecstatic emotional states, similar to those caused by other intense experiences such as orgasm or the creation of art, contact with nature, or a spiritual experience. Women experience a feeling of being one with what is taking place as in the fusion of the lover with the loved one, the mother and father with the child, the artist with the work being created. One transcends the ordinary, familiar sense of self, to achieve an extraordinary understanding of being one with the cosmos. Women sense their autonomy, at the same time they experience being part of all that is, ever has been, ever will be. These experiences move beyond ordinary time and space. Ego boundaries seem to dissolve. They are the states that we read about in mystical literature, and are accessible to each of us. This expansion and deepening of our personal awareness is one of the unexpected and wonderful aspects of having a baby. Psychologist Abraham Maslow called these sensations "peak experiences." We invite these states all too rarely, and therefore their manifestation can be unfamiliar and frightening at first.

It is my hope that knowledge of some of the emotional stages that an expectant mother will pass through during the year may help her to realize the peak aspects of pregnancy and birth, and minimize the troubling ones. In the second part of this chapter, we will look at the expectant father's experience of pregnancy.

Themes and Stages: Patterns to Work with

We are learning that the mother will move through predictable stages of development during the pregnancy, not only biologically, but psychologically and spiritually as well. The interrelationship of these levels is becoming increasingly clear. In the chart that follows, I have summarized some of the most dramatic of these changes as they are now understood to occur. Changes will not appear and disappear as abruptly as listed but these themes may be a useful guideline for your own individual reactions.

Emotions and Feelings During Pregnancy

First Three Months (first–twelfth week)

- Ambivalence, uncertainty even when pregnancy is planned
- Joy; pride in fertility
- Fear of incompetence, fear of harming the developing fetus
- Acceptance of pregnancy
- Vulnerability
- Loss of control; natural process is taking over
- Fear of dependency; concerns about trust
- Freedom in sex; heightened sexuality, no worry about contraception (occasionally fear of harming fetus during sex)
- Moodiness; unpredictability; increased awe in relation to the pregnant state, emotional sensitivity
- Increased need for love and affection

Second Three Months (thirteenth–twenty-four week)

- Increased dreams, fantasies; uncensored emotional reactions
- Introspection

- Heightened awareness of unconscious processes
- Sense of excitement and reality in experiencing "quickening" of baby; awareness of irreversibility of events
- Free-floating anxiety
- Thoughts about one's own mother; transition from daughter to mother, with accompanying conflicts and fears
- Shift in dependency from mother to husband

Third Three Months (twenty-fourth–fortieth week)

- Ambivalence towards changing body
- Pride in full-blown pregnancy; reveling in role of lifegiver (identification with divine aspects of motherhood, female goddess myths)
- Impatience with physical discomfort
- Need for affection and recognition of special state
- Fear of death; fear of letting go; fears about labor and delivery
- Fears of separation from the baby
- Need for security, resentment of dependency
- Fear of abnormality of baby
- Anxiety about maternal capability
- Discomfort with increased fetal activity and size; sense of being invaded
- Insomnia; awkwardness
- Nesting: excited preparation for baby's arrival, naming, fixing crib

Postpartum (Reintegration)

- Need for family bonding, mother-child bonding
- Need for affection, reassurance, praise, security
- Celebratory period
- Emotional swings due to worries about: competence in breast feeding, about mothering the baby, role as lover and partner
- New sense of identity needs personal integration
- Need for social reintegration with community

It is clear that the hormones of pregnancy affect a woman's

body as it makes a baby. Although one naturally anticipates and does not wish to resist these hormonally mediated physical changes, it is the effect of these hormones on her emotional state that a woman may be totally unprepared for and frightened by. In trying to maintain her equilibrium, she may resist the impetus towards the accompanying psychological changes that are preparing her for the totally new role as mother. In addition, hormonal changes that create an altered state—often a transcendent one— may be even more difficult to allow. However, instead of perceiving her feelings, dreams and fantasies as aberrant or "crazy," she can view this period as a positive source of new understanding of herself and her world. Consciously letting go—surrendering—to the gamut of changes can open her up to the possibility of real personal transformation.

The expectant mother is, undeniably, undergoing a crisis of transition. Everything in her life is changing. This crisis has a dual nature, representing both danger and opportunity. "Crisis," says Richard Grossman in *Choosing and Changing*, "can only be avoided by those who refuse to undertake the journey of becoming."

One frightening pattern during pregnancy is often a regressive return to earlier attitudes and modes of behavior. Even a woman who is mature and sure that she wants a child may find herself on an emotional seesaw, swinging from positive to negative feelings toward her pregnant state and her life in general. For example, she may normally accept the necessity of her partner's business trips but during pregnancy she may have a hard time with his absence, which may bring to the surface exaggerated childlike feelings of insecurity and abandonment. These irrational feelings may confuse and irritate her partner, who may be beset by his own anxieties about the impending financial responsibility of parenthood.

A pregnant woman may feel unpredictably wide fluctuations of mood, resulting in outbursts of laughter, unexplained anxiety, sudden tears, depression, fearful dreams, embarrassing vulnerability or the tendency to be superstitious. Both she and her partner may find this unfamiliar behavior disconcerting, to say the least.

Although many of a pregnant woman's fears may be projections into an unknown future, others are firmly based on the actual changes that are taking place in her daily life. For example, she may worry about her sexual attractiveness as her body swells, her changing relationship to her partner as they become a family and her imminent loss of independence as the caretaker of a tiny baby. The dependent aspects of pregnancy are already giving her intimations of this. Some of her anxiety centers, too, around the very new economic responsibility that is part of parenthood. These threads converge and weave together, adding to the sum of each partner's individual anxieties. Taken one by one or all together, these questions will profoundly disturb the normal rhythms of a couple's life. It becomes necessary to seek new ways of achieving balance and harmony. For example, a man may need to rearrange his schedule, as much as is feasible, in response to his partner's vulnerability at this time; a woman may need to reassure her partner that the baby is not pushing him aside. Reassurances to unspoken questions can be crucial to maintaining this important bond during a time when the self-images of both partners are threatened.

It is not unusual for a woman to feel ambivalent in the early months as she becomes aware of the awesome and irreversible responsibility that she is undertaking. Poet Judith Thurman writes:

I am appalled by the definiteness of motherhood. Once you have a child you are never, afterward, not a mother. It is as if you were the ocean and the child a continent that rises up in you—usurping your energy, attracting settlers and institutions, forcing you to become part of history.

Once having decided to become a parent, pregnancy is a "point of no return."

In Grete L. Bibring's ten-year studies of the psychological aspects of pregnancy, at Beth Israel Hospital in Boston, it was discovered that *all* women exhibited significant and far-reaching psychological changes when pregnant. It is apparent from the work of Bibring and others that there is a distinct pattern of *pregnancy consciousness*. Some women are thrown off balance more than others. And each woman's pregnancy is quite different from her previous one partially because she has been changed physiologically, but also because her social and psychological self-awareness is altered each time. Experienced nurses and midwives observe that mothers who seem to have it together during pregnancy frequently fly apart in the postpartum stage, often soon after birth. These health professionals feel that confronting emotions during pregnancy is crucial to the adjustment into parenthood. It is interesting to note that pregnant women who are referred to psychotherapists for help during the course of pregnancy appear to achieve striking therapeutic results. Therapists report that problems are close to the surface during this open and receptive time and can be handled in relatively few sessions. Although the content of such therapy may be similar to that presented by severely neurotic patients, who might need two years or more to confront the same material, it is handled far more directly and easily by pregnant women. Says Dr. Gerald Caplan of Harvard's School of Communy Health:

> All kinds of fantasies and needs and wishes, which were previously unconscious, are now allowed out into consciousness, without producing as much anxiety as you would expect. It is as though during this period, the ego, probably as a result of its increased strength due to metabolic changes, does not mind living with these previously unconscious appetites.
>
> Concepts of Mental Health

A crucial psychological theme during pregnancy is a woman's relationship to her own mother. The intimate dependency of her infancy and childhood has evolved into a more independent relationship during the course of her puberty, adolescence and young womanhood. At this point, the mother-daughter relationship reaches a plateau. Although both the positive and negative aspects of the old relationship may remain, the mother and daughter may be more distant—both emotionally and geographically. During pregnancy, a woman may long to resume the old dependent relationship with her family, particularly with her mother or a close female friend. Although she may not act on her feelings, the longing may be intense. Negative feelings may emerge also. The long-forgotten or suppressed feelings of love-hate based on early dependency reemerge during pregnancy to be faced once again. In her normal, introverted state around the time of quickening, her thoughts return to old unresolved feelings about her own mother. She may feel more loving or more rebellious or angrier about the frustrating relationship she has with her mother or may experience all these feelings simultaneously. She can progress in her own evolution by confronting these feelings head on, assisted by the powerful dynamics of her own biochemistry. Pregnancy becomes an opportunity to move through this dependent stage to one in which the daughter sees herself as coequal with her mother. As the daughter, she can begin to see herself as a separate and distinct person and a potentially capable mother in her own right. This realization can bring her closer to accepting her mother as a distinct person as well.

Before the birth, in essence, the expectant mother belongs to her family of origin—after the birth, she establishes her own family. In other cultures, prescribed behavior helps guide mothers and daughters through the transition. These traditional patterns of behavior acknowledge a need for the familiarity, wisdom and support of one's own mother. In India, for example, a Punjab girl leaves her husband and her mother-in-law, with whom she may still feel shy, and travels to the home of her birth to be with her own mother and the village midwife, whom she has known throughout her life. Contemporary women are no less in need of traditional guidance, expertise and emotional support to alleviate their fears of this unknown and unpredictable period.

Questions of "Who am I?" arise quite normally during this

period. Who am I in relation to my changing body and the being growing inside me? Who am I in relation to my mother who brought me to life? Moving from simply being daughter to a stage where being a mother is the predominant focus brings to the surface a sense of identification with the mythological mother figures: earth goddesses and the Universal, or Divine, Mother.

In the last three months, there are the joyful, practical tasks of preparation for the birth itself and the baby's arrival: attending childbirth classes, lining a bassinet, painting a room. Underlying the outward-directed tasks is the necessary accompanying emotional preparation which goes on at the same time in unconscious forms—in dreams and fantasies working just below her daily level of consciousness.

Some of the anxiety naturally centers around the well-being of each member of the family. A woman may be anxious about injury to herself and may even fantasize about her own death, or be obsessed with fear that a serious accident or unknown danger will befall her partner, or that the baby will be abnormal, die during delivery or be stillborn. These concerns often progress in galloping fashion, often activated by the reading of a newspaper account of a disaster or watching TV news.

The normal anxieties of pregnancy are further aggravated by cultural messages absorbed in childhood. In fact, for generations, women have been raised with tales of the risks of long, difficult and painful labors, maternal death in childbirth and strange infant anomalies and birth injuries. Of course, there can be complications in childbirth, but it is important to remember that ninety-five percent of all births are normal. Deaths and injuries are rare.

Some of a woman's fears are primitive, even primordial—arising from the deeper recesses of the psyche, and difficult to explain in a contemporary context. Periodically, during pregnancy, some women may feel that their happiness arouses the envy of the gods and spirits, recalling from their childhood the myths and fairy tales of supernatural beings who inflict harm on mothers and their children: the malevolent, wicked witch in Rapunzel, for instance, in Grimm's *Fairy Tales,* who lures the baby away. Even today, as in earlier times, inconsistent as it may be with our rational training, superstitious relatives and friends warn the pregnant mother that the "evil eye" will bring trouble. Psycho-analyst Helene Deutsch speaks of these primitive fears in *The Psychology of Women:*

> In the educated woman of our own civilization, the feeling is an "irrational sensation". . . . Fantasies of monsters and unnatural births disturb the joy of expectation and fill the pregnant woman with anxieties. These are typical and found all over the world; women who have never been superstitious develop superstitions, fears of magic forces, etc.

Fears of death and dying often fascinate and obsess pregnant women. They may read newspaper articles about the death of someone or be frightened by a program seen on TV.

Dreams of death occur often. In fact, pregnant women dream about death more frequently than their nonpregnant friends—forty percent as compared to ten percent. In the last phase of pregnancy, typical dreams and fantasies may concern losing the baby or having it delivered in a bizarre way. These dreams and fantasies can be quite frightening. Some women dream that they destroy their child or throw their baby out the window: "I had a dream that after I had my baby, I forgot all about it. I didn't feed it for days—it started to get smaller and died."

Or they are concerned about how the baby will get out: "How is a person twenty-one inches long going to get out of me?"

The anxieties and fears take many forms. Early in pregnancy, a woman may be afraid that she will lose the baby; later on, she may fear that her partner will abandon her or die and leave her alone and helpless. Intimately as they are involved with the crea-tion of new life, it is not surprising that they are poignantly aware of its possible end.

Not only are pregnant women close to their own unconscious process, but they appear to be connected to the deepest levels of the collective unconscious. Their fantasies and dreams probably serve to guide them through the profound psychological and transpersonal changes that this passage in the life cycle involves. The psyche works in mysterious and wondrous ways. If the concern and fascination with death is seen as an expanded awareness of continuous transition and of the polarities of the life experience—of life and death—the awesome fantasies, phobias and fears can be explored and understood in quite a different dimension—as an opportunity for deeper insight into one's own life process, instead of as a crisis.

Most subtle of all is the sense that one's psychic self is dying—the old self giving way to the new parent self. Both men and women share these fears. It is partly the subconscious process of surrendering the old self, rather than a morbid obsession with dying, that activates symbols of death and subsequent rebirth in dreams and waking consciousness. These symbolic dreams may allow us to reach beyond our unique personal experience to touch the mystical levels of a wider human experience, enabling us to dissolve the ego boundaries which separate us from each other.

It is this transpersonal aspect of childbearing that is so little discussed. Grof speaks of it. Psychologist Rollo May discusses this sense of oneness and the fears that surround intimacy in *Love and Will*, as he speaks of orgasm

> as a psychophysical symbol of the capacity to abandon one's self, to give up present security in favor of the leap towards the deeper experience—the known for the unknown. It is not by accident that the orgasm often appears symbolically as death and rebirth.

In orgasm, in deep union with our polar opposite, there is surrender. If only for seconds, one experiences the absence of ego boundaries, the loss of self. In Bali, in fact, the act of making love is called "becoming one." By virtue of sexual union, in the act of love, each time, we are renewed. We *are* changed. As May has written:

* * *

When we love, we give up the center of ourselves. We are thrown from our previous state into a void; and though we hope to attain a new world, a new existence, we can never be sure. . . . We give, and give up our own center; how shall we know that we will get it back?

During pregnancy, a woman literally and symbolically has these longings and fears. The symbiosis with the baby is an experience of union for her and reminiscent of her own gestation period in the womb. As May points out, this earliest period of union is repeated in adult life in sexual union:

The sexual act is the most powerful enactment of relatedness imaginable, for it is the drama of approach and entrance and full union, then partial separation . . . then a complete reunion again. It cannot be an accident of nature that in sex we enact the sacrament of intimacy and withdrawal, union and distance, separating ourselves and giving in full union again.

It is *not* an accident; it is the reiteration of an earlier relationship each of us had with our mothers. Deeply engrained in our memory is this archetypal theme, from which myths and fairy tales derive.

On the other side of ecstasy in love is awareness of death and just as in the ecstatic lovemaking between a man or a woman, so too, in the midst of the pleasure of the symbiotic ecstasy of mother-love, pregnant women often fear that merging with the baby may destroy the self.

Confronting these deep arcane levels of the psyche allows a woman to experience the primordial process of change as she moves from merely being the child to her mother to becoming the mother to her child as well. Death and rebirth. Allowing the old self to die and a new self to be reborn to a new level in the unfolding spiral of her life—as a mother.

Perhaps it is the gathering intensity of mother-love that readies a woman for bonding and that also at the same time evokes the fear of symbolic death in the immediate separation. She realizes that the baby she has nurtured and cradled within her body for nine long months must now be surrendered. There is anxiety connected with these feelings of separation, even though she may feel ready for the pregnancy to be over and know that in losing the "fetus," she is gaining a child.

There may even be the poignant sense that as she loses the baby within her, the child is also losing her. The relationship must change. The harmony between mother and child is broken; the nine-month symbiosis is over; each one of them must adjust to their new state. A Jungian analyst describes the following dreams reported by a pregnant patient two weeks before her baby was born. In the first, she was in heaven and had to practice a gliding motion in order to return to earth. Though she knew landing on earth meant death, she was forced to let go. She landed, died and then awoke. Later, she had another dream in which she was moving up and down on the waves of the ocean and was commanded to surrender to the movement of the waves. This dream prepared her for the later surrender in childbirth.

Changing sexual needs and feelings are a major concern for a woman and her partner during the childbearing year.

Our feelings about ourselves as sexual beings obviously cannot be separated from the sum total of our feelings and needs and attitudes, but during pregnancy a woman may experience new and unfamiliar intensities of sexual rhythms. These hormonally stimulated changes may seem random and frightening, causing her to feel that her sexual identity is wildly fluctuating and unpredictable. Her sexual self-image may be threatened as a result. These feelings may range from a dismaying lack of interest in sex to bewildering, all-consuming erotic feelings. It is not unsual for a woman in this state to walk down the street imagining that everyone knows how sexy she's feeling.

In general, during the first pregnancy, Masters and Johnson's studies show a decrease in interest and sexual performance in the first trimester, but an increase in erotic feeling in the second trimester. In fact, eighty percent of the women questioned by them reported greater sexual satisfaction then, compared both to the earlier months of pregnancy, and to their experience before pregnancy.

A little-discussed fact is that many of the physiological changes which normally occur during sexual arousal when a woman is not pregnant—such as increased blood supply in the genital region, increased vaginal lubrication, tension and erection of breasts and nipples, tilting of the uterus—are normal phenomena of the pregnant state. Thus, it may be, as Libby Colman and Elisabeth Bing suggest in their book, *Sex During Pregnancy*, that pregnant women may feel more or less "turned on" all the time. In addition, pleasure may be enhanced when lovemaking is no longer affected by the need for contraception. These unusually intense and unfamiliar feelings of constant arousal may also be a source of anxiety to a woman and her partner; desire for frequent sex may be interpreted as excessively demanding or "needy" behavior. Expectant fathers also go through a spectrum of sexual fantasies and feelings of their own during this period. Watching his partner's body change and grow, month by month, provides dramatic proof to the expectant father that an irreversible transformation is taking place. A women's visible fertility may create many conflicting reactions in her partner: jealousy over her natural lifegiving productivity, fear of the Madonna she has become (and guilt at desiring a virginal Madonna figure), concern about entering her "already-occupied" body. Depending on his own background and self-esteem, this may temporarily wreak sexual havoc with his potency and his feelings of adequacy. Whether he turns to another woman for reassurance and sex or only thinks about doing so, his neediness may make him feel both guilty and resentful at the same time. This can create distance just when a couple needs to be most supportive of each other. On the positive side, a man may also be drawn into a nurturing role and become a thoughtful caretaker of his partner and of the developing baby. This, too, however, may have its complications, for his new caretaking impulses may frighten him, since his experience as a man in this culture has probably not encouraged him to develop this aspect of himself.

At the beginning of pregnancy, the lack of interest in sex may stem from morning sickness, fears of miscarriage, or just plain fatigue. If sex is the main form of physical expression of love between partners, a woman may feel deprived of the physical touching she needs during this vulnerable time. Fondling, caressing, massaging each other are other ways to express loving and sexual feelings; it is crucial to begin to explore alternative ways to give pleasure to each other. Recent books on sexuality can help a couple express and fulfill their individual needs (see Bibliography). A man's awareness of his pregnant partner's increased needs for tenderness, affection and care can significantly reduce tensions and avoid a retreat into resentful distance. What affects the mother affects the baby and, just as importantly, may influence the future relationship between mother and child. Psychologist Dr. Gerald Caplan of Harvard stresses:

We all know that a woman needs increased vitamins and proteins during pregnancy, and that if she doesn't get these she is likely to have all kinds of difficulties and complications. In just the same way, she needs increased supplies of love and affection and if she does not get them, she may have difficulty in giving love and affection to her child.

Affection, cuddling and lovemaking, if viewed in this light, are ways to nurture everyone involved; mother, father and child. It is, as the Yurok Indians believe, a way to teach love and tenderness in the womb. Rather than being seen as an increased demand on the expectant father, it gives him an essential, nurturing role.

Near the end of the pregnancy, most women feel needy and dependent, as do many men. Women are apt to be self-involved, introspective, consumed with the complexity of what is happening inside their bodies. Some are anxious. Many are just plain uncomfortable.

A woman's lack of interest in sex, coupled with her increased irritability, may strain her partner's empathy to its limits. The anxiety about the now very imminent birth, in the absence of a tender way.to release tension, can build up to a potentially explosive situation. It is essential to be able to talk openly about what's happening. A couple's reluctance or inability to discuss the problem does not deny its importance. Honest exchange about the most intimate of human encounters is an art that few of us are skilled at. So much seems at stake. Doctors may not be able to provide the needed solutions and it may be wise to talk to friends, in addition to reading about the ways in which others have successfully developed new ways of relating.

How a woman responds to the changes of pregnancy will vary according to individual sexual appetite, family attitudes carried along from childhood and the impact of cultural myths, taboos and superstitions. It is surprising to see how pervasive and influential these myths and taboos can be. They seem to be almost as powerful now in the '80s as they have been in preliterate cultures.

During pregnancy, when each partner's self-image is undergoing a change from person to the role of "parent," both partners need extra reassurance. She needs to know she is still attractive to him; he needs to know he is not being replaced by the person in the womb. A woman's view of herself and the transformation she is undergoing, of which her body is a visible manifestation, form part of the psychological climate of the baby's experience in the womb and during birth. Far from being supported and affirmed as she moves from adolescence to womanhood to motherhood, and later to menopause, a woman often has to struggle to learn about herself, about what's happening biologically, as if the workings of her body are an unmentionable, mysterious secret best concealed. Advances made in the field of women's health, as a result of the women's movement, fortunately are making available to all women information about their psychology and biology that will help them make intelligent decisions in their lives.

A woman's sense of herself as a sexual person is delicate and constantly shifting throughout her life, in ways that men do not experience so acutely. During pregnancy in particular, her body image, confidence in her sexual attractiveness and her sense of identity as a woman-person in the outer world are the focus of many conflicts throughout the nine months.

As the actual birth approaches, many emotions intensify. The pregnant couple is as close to the presence of life as to the possibility of death. In addition, the birth itself may have powerful sexual overtones reminiscent of the "letting go" and fear of death in orgasm. Women and men may find themselves suspended on an edge where their sense of life and death is enormously heightened. Actor Donald Sutherland has vivid memories of the birth of his two children, at which he assisted:

> They were the best two days of my life. It is a very sexual thing to be right there when your child is being born. You just want to make love. It's as simple as that. But I don't plan on having any more children. In a strange way, seeing the two kids born was like psychologically participating in my own death . . . and I don't want to feel that again. It was like a part of me was cut away to give birth to a new life.
> San Francisco *Chronicle*,
> September 30, 1979

We are unused to perceiving or talking about the sexuality of birth. Generally, it has been a taboo subject. Only recently have women begun to share openly their feelings of pleasure and sexual arousal during birth and nursing. Acknowledging these natural feelings can increase the mutual pleasure and well-being of mother and child. Mr. Sutherland's description of his reaction to the births of his children is a fascinating illustration of the complex emotions birth can evoke in fathers, too—a sense of mortality, coupled with heightened sexuality. Indeed, the parents who are bringing life into the world may themselves feel an intensified sense of *being alive*.

During the pregnant year, as a man becomes a father, he may feel:

- Things will never be the same again.
- She'll love the baby more than me.

- She'll not desire me again.
- I won't be a good father.
- Nothing I do satisfies her.
- We made a baby!
- Her full breasts and her round belly turn me on.
- I can't understand the feelings she describes.
- I'll never be as important to the baby as she is.
- I envy her ability to create a person in her body.
- I love her sexual energy.
- I feel trapped.
- I feel left out.
- I can't wait to show off my kid.
- I'm afraid she won't be able to stand the pain. What if she screams for drugs?
- I won't be able to make enough money for all of us.
- I'm afraid she'll die.
- I don't want to end up as a diaper changer. It's demeaning.
- This is more important than anything else I've ever done.

Until recently, most books on the pregnant years mentioned the father as the donor of the sperm on page one and promptly dismissed him. A typical book, *Expectant Motherhood*, focuses entirely on the mother, as though the father had no role except the genetic one. The situation has changed, fortunately. Fathers are becoming involved in preparation for parenthood. Although they have been encouraged to participate actively at the time of labor and delivery, little attention has been focused on their emotional needs during the year preceding the baby's birth. If we can tap the psychological resources of the father, says psychiatrist Dr. Arthur Colman, he can be a deep well of support. However, we must also understand and meet his needs. In the '70s Dr. Colman and others have been studying attitudes of expectant fathers and mapping the psychological stages that men pass through during the pregnant year.

Dr. James Herzog of the Harvard Medical School shows us that patterns of psychological experience in expectant fathers are as mappable as those of expectant mothers. These stages are not keyed to predictable physiological changes in men's bodies, but they are present and observable. We have simply never taken formal notice of these changes. Despite the fact that all men may not exhibit them to the same degree, "certain themes, feelings and concerns" repeat themselves across the pregnant months and are related to those of their partners. All men, however, are not in touch with their feelings to the same degree. Herzog found that the fathers who were most aware of their own feelings about the pregnancy were those men who were "most attuned" or sympathetic to their partners' intense feelings. He observed that the deeper the intimacy and commitment between partners, the easier it was for a man to fully participate in the changes that pregnancy brings. Furthermore, he found that the origins of a father's nurturing behavior went back to a man's own childhood. In couples where intimacy and commitment were weaker, concerns and fantasies about fathering were blurred or nonexistent.

The most empathetic fathers spoke of the difference between simply having sex and "making a baby." When the conception was confirmed, these men were delighted: "Making the kid was a high," "We felt an inner glow," "I've got the cock that made her pregnant . . . my seed is sown." One man felt it gave him a reason for being. All were pleased with their potency and excited by the idea of creating a new life. The couples whose relationships were not as close, in contrast, did not plan the conception together, and in fact, some of these women chose not to share the news of their pregnant state for a while.

Toward the end of the first trimester, the fathers who were most involved reported that their fantasies during lovemaking changed; that they experienced a shift in their inner life. Indeed, reports Herzog, it was through their sexual activity that they got in touch with their conflicts and feelings about caretaking and moved to a deeper understanding of their masculinity.

The sex lives of many men improved after their partners conceived. They not only wanted to be more loving toward their partners but they were able to ask them for love more easily. For some, odd fantasies emerged during lovemaking. For example, there was a feeling of "refertilizing the pregnancy." Not only were they giving to the mother but to the baby as well. Some imagined they were "the breast" or "huge bottles of milk." One remarked, "They need more and I have it to give." For some fathers, it was a pleasure to have these new feelings; others felt irritation and concern about their capacity to meet the increased sexual demands.

Some of the fathers were preoccupied with getting nurtured through sexual activity and often felt deprived. Just as pregnant women need love and affection, so the men also may need extra evidence that they are still loved and desired.

In mid-pregnancy, a man who is empathetic with his partner's experience may be far more conscious of his own insides. Manifestations of "couvade" symptoms were shown by virtually everyone in Herzog's study. The *couvade* is such a fascinating phenomenon that it is worth examining in some detail. It is a psychosomatic expression of a psychological need that has only recently been rediscovered.

Couvade, derived from the old French word *couver* meaning to brood or to hatch, is a folk tradition that has been practiced with many variations in many parts of the world, and is of two types: 1) the father's imitation of the mother's role during and after childbirth, and 2) the subjection of the father to various dietary restrictions and to other privations and duties, often unpleasant, in order to protect the mother and baby from evil. Reports of the *couvade* date back to Herodotus, who discovered it in Africa, and to Marco Polo, who encountered it in ancient China.

The custom of *couvade* shows up in many societies today. No one seems to know its origin or understand its meaning fully. One mythical version of the origin of the *couvade*, according to feminist author Helen Diner, is an Irish legend which tells of the pregnant wife of Crunniuc, who was forced to run a race against horses. Immediately after winning, she gave birth to twins. In the agonies of her birth pangs, she condemned all men who heard her cries to suffer the pains of childbirth for four days and five nights. The curse carried through nine generations. Many theories exist about the origin of *couvade*. Some think the custom arose to help the father identify with the new child and to accept responsibility

for it. Since it is practiced almost exclusively in matriarchal societies, it may have been created to indicate that the act of birth is
far more important than the act of insemination, and that it is
only through the ritualized enactment of "giving birth" that the
male becomes a father. Still other theories suggest the *couvade*
may be an attempt to allow the father a more significant role
through the psychodramatic technique of role reversal, or that it is
an attempt to share the pain of childbirth through sympathetic
magic.

Before, during, or after confinement, the father acts out the
birth by lying in his bed, like his laboring wife. He moans, writhes,
sobs and is nursed attentively. He accepts food restrictions for
days or weeks before and after the birth occurs and is subject to
the same customs as is the mother. For example, he is considered
unclean after the birth until he has taken his first bath.

The practice has been observed recently by anthropologists in
places as widespread as Siberia, the Malay Archipelago, in various
countries in Africa and in Brazil and India. Somatic symptoms of
couvade are reported in studies today in the United States. Often
men express hidden feelings and will react physically to their
partner's pregnancy. Some men notice their breasts swelling or
sense a feeling of fullness. Sometimes, when a woman feels her
partner is negative about the pregnancy, her attacks of nausea and
fatigue may increase. On the other hand, if her partner is more
strongly motivated towards parenthood and she is the more conflicted one, he may have the "morning sickness" and exhibit
vicarious involvement through symptoms of pregnancy such as
fatigue, dizziness, nausea, a swelling belly or breasts, food cravings, even weight gain. These "*couvade*" responses are not at all
uncommon.

In each society, the father's role is handled differently. In
egalitarian societies, he is a valued and supportive participant, as
in Polynesia, where attitudes and practices are wholesomely simple, unburdened by complicated ritual and customs and sex roles
are quite equal. In such societies, there is no *couvade*. On the
other hand, in male-dominated societies, where pregnancy is considered a dangerous time for the community at large and the

pregnant woman is viewed as dirty and polluting, she is segregated and he is restrained from the role of an involved supporter. Even in female-dominated societies, a pregnant woman will be supported by other women and fathers will be excluded. In these societies, the father will engage in *couvade* practices or participate vicariously.

In Java, it is believed that the husband's presence hastens delivery, since the child longs for its father, and therefore it is important that he attend the birth. Immediately after the birth, the mother and newborn baby bathe in the river, and thereafter the mother resumes her normal activities. The father, however, goes to bed, pretends to be sick and takes over the postpartum confinement while his wife prepares special food for him. (It is clear that *couvade* has its disadvantages for the woman!)

Anthropologist Margaret Mead's analysis of *couvade* practice links it to "birth envy" in males. The work of Melanie Klein, a psychoanalyst, speaks of male envy in relation to the creativity of women in childbirth. In fact, some psychologists say that a pregnant woman expects that envy and a dread of it creates anxiety in her. Bruno Bettleheim claims that a man who envies his partner's childbearing ability is not able to show sympathy for her. He expects, if not compels, her to resume her work immediately after childbirth although she may be exhausted and need to recuperate. The man, says Bettleheim, as husband and father, is permitted to rest. (Instead of sympathy, emphasizes Bettleheim, the father insists on the special care for himself that would be appreciated by her but that he denies her. Bettleheim concludes that the expression of birth envy is less likely in a male-dominated society.) He suggests that both male initiation rites and *couvade* rituals are parallel to a woman's childbirth rituals.

There are many other psychological phenomena experienced by men during the second trimester.

During the middle period of the pregnancy, both Herzog and Colman believe, men relive a childhood stage involving the hermaphroditic fantasy in which a boy believes he can both fertilize and bear a child. Colman reports that expectant fathers' dreams are filled with images of bearing and delivering babies. The appearance of these images in dreams, rather than being embarrassing, is a healthy sign that men are acknowledging their envy and passing beyond it. Just as for women, if these often unconscious feelings are not dealt with by the expectant fathers during pregnancy, they can reemerge at a later time in negative ways.

At this time, men began to perceive themselves as playing dual sexual roles. In Herzog's studies, the fathers who were most intimate with their partners wanted to play at being both male and female. Many empathetic fathers, in fact, introduced variations in their lovemaking that allowed them to "feel penetrated at the same time that they were penetrating." These men felt that sexual activity made the baby happy and healthy. Others were either concerned that they might hurt the baby during sex, or that "the baby might bite." When a couple's personal relationship was warm and open, most men felt that the sexual relationship reflected this and was equally good. Toward the end of the pregnancy, reactions might be similar to that of one man who felt the mother's body was a "house" for the baby, which he couldn't enter.

Some men find the swelling belly to be sensual, a turn-on; others feel embarrassed and put off by the physical changes in their partner's body and will avert their eyes. This awkwardness can create a personal distance. However, expectant mothers who feel unattractive and become jealous during pregnancy may find it reassuring to know that men, by and large, are more pleased by their partner's pregnant body than the women themselves are.

Some men unconsciously identify with the baby and the time they themselves were growing inside their mother's body, and may feel threatened. Others have been conditioned to consider the pregnant body unerotic. Women themselves may transmit this message because of the negative image they've encountered in the media.

This whole complex of psychosexual feelings is the harbinger of important change. What follows in mid-pregnancy, for men as well as for women, is an increased pressure to resolve one's relationship to one's own parents. This urge arises even if not recognized or acted on.

Interestingly, Herzog found that just as expectant mothers needed to rework previous conflicts and unresolved feelings with their parents of the same sex, so too expectant fathers have a need to work out aspects of their own father-son relationship. Previous conflicts and tension come into play, particularly in relation to a man's own father. It appears to be one of the necessary psychological steps towards achieving maturity. Herzog says that almost every involved father attempted to straighten things out with his father, often with his wife's help. Although these attempts were not always completely successful, relations improved as a result of the effort. Herzog observes that men who were least successful in breaking through these old barriers had the most difficult time during the second half of the pregnancy. Most knew that the process was important in some way. "How I hook up with my old man determines how the kid will hook up with me." It is as if men, like women, are symbolically and specifically trying to make a developmental leap from being the child of their fathers to becoming fathers to their child.

Colman discusses the same issue with a slightly different emphasis, feeling that it is difficult for fathers to fully participate in the pregnancy—for there is nothing comparable they can do. It *is* an opportunity, however, for men to get in touch with the feminine—receptive—side of their nature and experience it. The pregnant year can be viewed as a demonstration of the interaction of opposites in the universe, a time to understand one's androgynous nature.

There are many psychological strands. Some expectant fathers become competitive with their partners, provoked by unresolved feelings of sibling rivalry with the unborn baby, first initiated at the birth of their own brothers or sisters. This may also happen when men become partners with women in *any* situation, such as a business partnership. There may also be residual memories of the separation at birth from their own mothers. A man may find that these and other primitive fears are hard to assimilate into the rational context in which he has functioned during his life up to this time.

Many men move on to the third trimester of the pregnancy

with concerns and feelings that are similar to their partner's. They too experience the mystery and magic surrounding the awesome event—a process that is larger than themselves or any one person, and know it to be beyond their ability to control. They too become more concerned with practical matters, realizing that it is a time to get one's house in order, both literally and figuratively. Men become interested in how others cope; how others raise their children. A caretaking sensibility comes into reality for these men. Intrusive fantasies also lessen with the decline of sexual activity. An outer-directed view replaces the absorption with the inner exploration of previous months. "It's out of my hands. I've done what I could. Now nature has to take its course."

It is fascinating to me that the theme of mystery and magic which appears in every culture was reiterated over and over in Herzog's study. The spectrum varied from an emphasis on the sinister (meaning left, intuitive) to an emphasis on the sublime (meaning inspiring awe, or below the threshold of conscious perception). Men began to sense the transpersonal dimensions of the experience of creation. There also emerged in fathers a more defined sense of the differences between male and female roles. And with that comes a new and deeper appreciation of their value as a person who goes out into the world, and conversely a new respect for the very particular bond between mother and child. There emerged a clearer view of his role as a male person in the family.

The psychological and social dynamics of pregnancy appear to be different for men and women. Reactions will vary, of course, reflecting upbringing, adult personality and individual circumstances. For a man in particular, since his psychological state during this period is not linked to metabolic changes, his experience and involvement will be more directly related to his personal history, his past difficulties and the way he has previously resolved conflicts.

Pregnancy, especially the first time, is a profound and often overwhelming experience for most women. All that they know and trust about themselves and their lives is called into question—

daily, in fact, many times each day for nine months! In turn, her partner is sharing her concerns, as well as having to cope with his own changes. How can this period of profound physiological and psychological change be made easier? Is it simply a passage to be endured in isolation, hoping for the best, or can acknowledgment of the distinct stages of pregnancy as current research now defines them give insights that place the transitional crisis in manageable perspective? Even further, could talking about these feelings, fears and hopes with other pregnant couples provide a sustaining foundation on which to develop as parents of a new family? Grete Bibring was one of the most articulate advocates in America for the potential usefulness of the support groups that are the subject of this book. Unfortunately, her ideas, communicated to other professionals in the late 1950s, have still not become part of routine prenatal care. Others, like Sheila Kitzinger, author and childbirth educator, have also advocated these ideas since then. Based on my experience with pregnant couples in the groups I have led, there is still an urgent need for such workshops, as a complement to the recent resurgence of interest in making the delivery itself more "natural" for both mother and child. In 1959, Bibring pointed out some telling paradoxes concerning our tendency to overemphasize the obstetric aspects of pregnancy and birth. In the 1980s, the warning still applies:

> Pregnancy, like puberty or menopause, is a period of crisis involving profound psychological as well as somatic change. As the modern family becomes isolated, and as other important group memberships break down, the individual must rely increasingly on the nuclear family, especially on the marital relationship, and this unit is rarely equipped to replace all these figures in their varied supportive functions.
>
> With increasing emphasis on the "scientific" in our society, less and less attention is paid to the unscientific, the irrational, the emotional and spiritual dimensions of human existence. The question may be raised here, then,

whether the enormous improvement in medical management, in lessening the physical dangers of pregnancy, has also contributed to a waning concern with the concomitant psychodynamics of this period.

There is then a lack of psychological understanding and support from the enlightened environment, and we see often exaggerated attempts on the part of the expectant mother to adjust consciously to the scientific viewpoints of pregnancy and its management. . . . What was once a crisis, with carefully worked out traditional customs of giving support to the woman passing through this crisis period, has become at this time a crisis with no mechanisms within the society for helping the woman involved in this profound change. . . . If this be so, then the importance of appropriate psychological care as part of the prenatal program becomes obvious. . . .

We may have to direct our attention to the period of pregnancy itself and find adequate ways to bring the psychological support in line with the achievements of today's obstetrics.

> Grete L. Bibring,
> Some Considerations of the
> Psychological Processes in
> Pregnancy

Since, as Bibring and Herzog point out, many of the superstitious customs surrounding pregnancy through the ages are no longer helpful to the modern pregnant couple in channeling and coping with the intense emotions that accompany pregnancy, what can we provide as a substitute, as a starting point that establishes common ground for pregnant couples?

What really happens to expectant parents during this period? What is provoked during the crisis? What is a positive environment for this juncture?

In 1972, I was absorbed by the question of how I might best help future parents examine their way of life as it affected the developing family. The answer for me turned out to be a series of Birth Workshops that I designed for pregnant couples, in which we would explore the social and psychological dynamics and the physical elements of the birth environment.

During pregnancy and childbirth, both parents have the potential to expand their previous understanding of their world. As other cultures have before us, we are finally recognizing that the process of becoming parents is a profound transitional crisis in family development—a period with characteristic patterns of development—a rite of passage which heralds a new stage for everyone involved. Honoring this time and acknowledging the feelings and emotional conflicts that it presents might enable parents to celebrate this important turning point instead of fearing or denying it.

Writer Ken Wilbur has said, "Crisis is an unfamiliar level of excitement." My goal was to make the unfamiliar familiar and to allow parents to transform this period of crisis into one of opportunity.

If the thought, the money, the religious enthusiasm, now expended for the regeneration of the race, were wisely directed to the generation of our descendants, to the conditions and environments of parents and children, the whole face of society might be changed before we celebrate the next centennial of our national life.

If there is a class of educators who need special education for their high and holy calling, it is those who assume the responsibility of parents. Shall we give less thought to the creation of an immortal being than the artist devotes to his statues or landscape? We wander through the galleries in the old world, and linger before the works of the great masters, transfixed with grace and beauty, the glory and the grandeur of the ideals that surround us; and with equal preparation, greater than these are possible in living, breathing humanity. The same thought and devotion in real life would soon give us a generation of saints, scholars, scientists, statesman; of glorified humanity; such as the world has not seen. To this hour, we have left the greatest event of life to chance . . .

A child's first right is to be well born of parents sound in body and mind. . . .

> from *Practical Housekeeping:*
> *A Careful Compilation of Tried and*
> *Approved Recipes, 1881*

IV

Loosening the Knots:
The Group Experience

Many people in different parts of the world
entertain a strong objection to having any knot
about their person at certain critical seasons,
particularly childbirth, marriage and death.
The Lapps think that a lying-in woman should
have no knots on her garments, because a knot
would have the effect of making the delivery
difficult and painful. In the East Indies, this
superstition is extended to the whole time of
pregnancy; the people believe that if a pregnant
woman were to tie knots, or braids, or make
anything fast, the child would thereby be con-
stricted or the woman herself be "tied up" when
her time came. Nay, some of them enforce the
observance of the rule on the father as well as
the mother of the unborn child.

In all these cases the idea seems to be that
the tying of a knot, would, as they say in the
East Indies, "tie up" the woman, in other
words, impede and perhaps prevent her
delivery, or delay her convalescence after the
birth.

In the island of Saghalien, when a woman is

in labor, her husband undoes everything that
can be undone. He loosens the plaits of his hair
and the laces of his shoes. Then he unties whatever is tied in the house or its vicinity. In the
courtyard, he takes the axe out of the log in
which it is stuck; he unfastens the boat, if it is
moored to a tree; he withdraws the cartridges
from his gun, and the arrows from his cross-
bow.

The same train of thought underlies a practice observed by some people of opening all
locks, doors and so on, while a birth is taking
place in the house. Among the Mandelings of
Sumatra, the lids of all chests, boxes, pans and
so forth are opened; and if this does not produce
the desired effects, the anxious husband has to
strike the projecting ends of some of the house-
beams in order to loosen them; for they think
that "everything must be loose and open to
facilitate the delivery."

Sir James Frazer,
The Golden Bough
1929

In the Birth Workshops, I hoped to create a concerned and supportive extended family and an emotionally safe environment. Conscious of the baby who was at the center of this change of state, I felt we might share together the profound changes that were taking place in each couple's sense of themselves, their feelings about each other and the ways in which their behavior might affect their unborn child.

By availing ourselves of the extraordinary sensitivity provoked by the hormonal changes of pregnancy, I hoped we might loosen the psychological knots and provide the support that was needed from the very beginning.

How was I to begin? I contacted couples through doctors, midwives, childbirth educators, friends, ads in *New York* Magazine and in the *Village Voice*, letting people know that I was conducting four-month-long workshops at no fee, as part of my doctoral research on the psychological and social aspects of the pregnant year. It was difficult to find people who were willing to spend the time and make the required time commitment. I wanted couples who would come once a week for four months; it was not to be a "drop-in" group. Finally, most group members were referred to me by friends or were people I encountered personally.

At times I despaired that the first group would never come

together. Pregnant women I met were intrigued, but many said, "*I'd* love to, but *he'd* never do it," or "I don't have the time." I was determined to have fathers as well as mothers. At dinner parties I got to be a bore, always inquiring about pregnant friends. Ultimately, my tenacity paid off. Seven couples signed up for the first group. One came through a woman I met at a party. Not pregnant herself but fascinated, she sent her brother and his pregnant wife. One couple came through *Ms.* Magazine friends, another through a male friend who couldn't have been less interested in birth. Two were sent by sympathetic obstetricians. The final couple read the ad in the paper. Seven pregnant couples—people who never would have met each other if not drawn together by their common interest in exploring pregnancy and birth. I was delighted. Unfortunately, a week before the first session, two couples had to drop out.

Despite this tentative beginning, the workshops were launched. Five couples joined me for the first session of the four-month-long venture. Much later, when the members of the first group had "graduated," other groups were organized, some meeting for many months, others for intensive weekends. The groups were usually small, numbering about ten men and women. This size allowed everyone to participate actively and yet was large enough to provide a variety of reactions and experience. In this chapter, I will present the reactions of one typical group as we met each week for several months.

The couples who participated in these support groups were, in general, white, middle class, primarily professionals—artists, writers, lawyers, architects, nurses, teachers—people who were intrigued by, though not particularly conscious of, the feelings provoked by the pregnancy. What they had in common was an interest in and a commitment to talking with others who were going through the same experience. There was a span of ages. Most of the couples were in their thirties, though a few were younger and some of the men were in their early forties. In the four-month-long support groups, all the couples were expecting their first child, but were at different stages of pregnancy. (One couple came even before they conceived.) In the groups that met only for one intense weekend, there was, generally, a mixture of first and second pregnancies. Most couples in all the groups chose "natural" or "prepared childbirth" as a method of delivery, committing themselves to participate jointly in prenatal training and all stages of labor and delivery. Some mothers were turned off by the idea of "natural childbirth." Instead, they were frankly eager to yield the responsibility of the delivery to their doctors, whom they had carefully chosen to make decisions for them. These women said they didn't care whether or not they were "knocked out" by drugs. Their attitude often changed, however, during the course of the workshop. In the last six weeks of their pregnancies, all of the couples were involved in other prenatal classes whose major focus was on preparation for labor and delivery *per se*.

I made it clear that my major interest and expertise were not in the obstetrical or medical aspects of birth, but that I thought it important for them to educate themselves in this area so that they could make informed choices about the kind of delivery they hoped to have—hospital or home, with or without anesthesia, etc. As the groups progressed, I would make clear my own preferences, and share my own experiences—details of my birth, and of the births of my three children. We all felt a strong sense of excitement as we embarked on exploring aspects of pregnancy that have been neglected or minimized in contemporary Western society. What began so long ago as an interest in defining what might be an optimum physical environment for giving birth developed into my conviction that the emotional and physical aspects of pregnancy and birth are inseparable.

At the beginning I conducted the groups alone; in the subsequent groups I worked with a male coleader. One of the coleaders was a physician, a father of four, whose practice of internal medicine was based on holistic principles. He had experience in mind-body therapies, such as bioenergetics, and in group techniques, and was especially interested in how family interactions affect psychological and physical health. Best of all, he was warm, loving and a sensitive listener. He was as enthusiastic as I, welcoming the opportunity to work with a normal, healthy life transition.

In the group setting, we hoped to create

* * *

- a safe place to raise questions and explore feelings—including expectations and fears;
- a supportive nonclinical environment in which parents-to-be shared their concerns with others moving through the same experience;
- ways to facilitate verbal and nonverbal communication in the couple relationship;
- insight and confidence in making personal decisions;
- tools, skills, information with which to design the birth experience;
- an atmosphere of celebration and joy.

When possible, I initiated the workshop with a two-day session held over a weekend, with couples returning home at night. Although this is ideal, it is not always feasible for people to spend two full days away from their everyday lives.

The sessions developed in both unstructured and structured ways. I experimented with explorative and supportive techniques that might help to make pregnancy a time of personal growth for each parent—as individuals, as a couple and as a part of a threesome, the developing family unit. I used awareness techniques that have been developed in the West over the past several decades, as well as ancient Eastern ones. Many I myself improvised as the group progressed. These exercises (see Chapter VIII) helped to bring to conscious awareness intense feelings and emotions, such as confusion, tenderness, ambivalence and dependency.

At the beginning of each session, I found it helpful to start with a warm-up exercise, which served effectively to dispel concerns accumulated during the day and to focus on any difficulties arising out of the pregnancy. Sometimes exercises were chosen to elicit feelings related to a particular theme. As trust developed in the group, so did spontaneity and expansiveness, and we were able to work in unstructured ways as well, allowing concerns to emerge spontaneously. Often a dramatic problem that had developed for one or another of the couples during the course of the week became the focus of the evening. On those evenings, role reversal might be used to highlight an issue that had arisen and thereby gain insight in a subjective way. For example, a man coming home from work may expect the cheerful attention he used to receive before the pregnancy; instead, he finds his partner moody, withdrawn, self-absorbed, or in need of emotional comforting. This discrepancy in their mutual needs can create feelings of rejection and explosive tension if what's happening isn't understood in a larger context. By taking each other's roles and playacting a typical incident, each partner may gain insights into the other's point of view. Group members can add their often valuable comments on the couple's behavior and point out unconscious behavior patterns. Since the workshop dealt with the shared concerns of pregnancy, problems discussed by one couple usually had significance for others.

On a warm Saturday in September 1972, my first group met at my home at ten in the morning for the first day of a two-day session. We gathered in the sunny living room of my garden apartment in New York City's Greenwich Village. We introduced ourselves, and talked about our expectations—positive and negative—for the group. I stated clearly that there were many things I hoped to learn along with them and that although I had a vague agenda, it was to be their group. I hoped the group would be responsive to their needs and their wishes would prevail. We had a preliminary discussion about time, schedules and commitment—details that in themselves are part of the process. Apprehensive and excited myself, I had to struggle with my own hopes, fears and expectations, along with everyone else. The couples were: Elena, a social worker, three months pregnant, and her husband, Dick, an architect; Rachel, a homemaker, not yet pregnant, and her husband, Alan, a resident in internal medicine; Amy, a weaver, four months pregnant, and her husband, Don, an economist; Ria, also about four months pregnant, a nursing student, and Eric, a teacher; Anne, a management consultant, three months pregnant, and her husband, Sam, an airlines executive. An interesting mix, everyone bringing his or her own particular life histories and attitudes to our work together.

Interestingly, as each couple described themselves briefly, no one mentioned their occupation. For the time being, at least, they simply identified with parenthood. Even Rachel and Alan, who had not yet conceived, chose that category. Positive reinforcement from the start. Encouraged by me, this couple had joined the group hoping that pregnancy might be "catching." They had tried everything else: she had been tested, he had been tested; they'd been through it all. We speculated that by focusing on the psychological process, the long-hoped-for conception might occur.

As we continued that morning, I suggested that each person keep a journal in which feelings, dreams, or important events would be recorded. So much was going to happen that it would be hard to recall it later if it were not written down.

I asked permission to videotape the sessions so that we would have a record for others and especially for my Ph.D. project. Several couples expressed concern that it would affect their ability to share intimately. Ria for one, didn't want to be recorded for "posterity"; others weren't sure what they felt. The decision was postponed until the end of the evening. Later, they all agreed that was fine, and we planned to start taping the next week.

The first exercise I introduced was a trust-building exercise called a blind walk: Everyone closes his-her eyes and allows him-herself to be guided wordlessly through the space, trusting that their partners will take care of them. They may lead each other up or downstairs, sit their partners down, guide them through different sound, temperature, and touch experiences—outside and inside the house. Simple as it seems, it is a surprisingly powerful and meaningful experience for pregnant couples in this increasingly interdependent time in their relationship. Symbolically, it is especially meaningful for a pregnant woman, who is involved in an organic experience, entrusting her body to others to guide her through.

Each couple had a turn leading and being led by their spouse and then working with another partner. Afterward, we discussed the experience together, sharing what had been learned about levels of trust. Several members talked about how much more secure they had felt with their spouses than with a stranger. Amy described the panic she felt as she was led around by a strange person; Don described the disorientation he felt when shifting light patterns penetrated his colored eyelids. Later that morning he realized how dependent he was on his partner in their life together, and how difficult it was for him to acknowledge it.

An exercise such as this one can provide unexpected insights into one's need for a secure, trusting relationship. Being able to depend on one's partner is an important foundation for being able to handle other relationships where trust is at stake: doctors, nurses, hospital personnel. The themes of trust and dependency recurred often during the four months we spent together. To all of us, it became apparent that during this vulnerable period each partner needs constant nurturing in order to expand and change. The relationship needs the same capacity to stretch as does the pregnant belly. Pregnant couples found that they had to be mother, father and family for each other. Often the demands made on each other were bound to feel excessive. The group began to provide additional emotional support.

After three hours of unfamiliar and stimulating interactions, everyone needed a break. We stopped to relax and share the pot luck meal that everyone had brought. "Breaking bread" together seemed an appropriate ritual for the nurturing process of exploration that we were embarking on, and it was also a chance to socialize on a more informal basis. Everyone gathered round the table in my country-style kitchen. The autumn sun filtered through the garden out back, creating golden stripes on polished floorboards. Graced with heavy rafters and a large fireplace, the kitchen had fed many families since it was built in 1835; its warm environment enhanced our workshop. It was an atmosphere that could not have been achieved at a prenatal clinic. Although no one had specifically designated what should be brought to the pot luck, the bread, salads and casseroles all came together as a three-course meal. Have you ever noticed how often things work out when one doesn't try to maintain control? It was as if from the beginning of our first session, we became a functioning organism. It was a joy to see the pregnant women survey the food-laden table. The men also beamed in anticipation, but they weren't feasting for two. Being well fed, however, increases everyone's feeling of well-being. Each couple brought food that was an expression of their life and attitudes: simple health food from one, complicated gourmet sauces and wine from another. We were already learning about each other.

After lunch, we gathered again and I asked them to participate in another exercise.

Meditation on Birth

In a room emptied of furniture, I asked everyone to lie down and form a mandala shaped like the spokes in a wheel, with their heads touching in the middle of the circle, husband and wives alternating as they lay on the floor. I began,

> Pay attention to your breathing. Simply allow its normal rhythm without controlling it. Relax more deeply with each breath—as it moves in and out, inhale and exhale— and with each breath let go of your thoughts, let them float by as you breathe out, let go of your persona, your profession, your attachments, just become aware of your breath connecting you to the universe.

After some minutes of stillness, I continued by guiding them back to the room and to their connection with each other. Then each couple was asked to join hands and with their eyes still closed to sense their partner's breathing rhythm and to breathe in unison with one another and with the baby in the womb.

> Get in touch with the rhythm you are now sharing, the rise and fall of joint breath . . . and with the baby's rhythm. . . . When you feel in rapport with each other, begin to meditate on the word "*birth*." Allow your

thoughts to arise and flow through your consciousness, let them come and go. Simply observe without trying to hold on to them, allow them to drift through. . . . When you are ready, open your eyes.

All of this took about twenty minutes. Quietly, still in meditative silence, we returned to the other room. Interestingly, some couples felt relaxed, chose new places to sit, but remained as a pair, however, in whatever place they resettled. Sometime later, when we discussed our seating patterns, couples became aware of how little time they had with each other during the week, and realized that it was not only for security in this unfamiliar situation that they chose to sit next to their partners, but in order to be able to be close and to touch.

We talked about what had happened that morning. Ria began:

I was aware of many new sensations in my body that I don't normally take time to sense. . . . It has changed. Rather than feeling uncomfortable about that, as I normally do, I was really digging it . . . and then I began to picture the development of the baby. I was acutely aware that my baby isn't ready to be born yet. I can't explain how I know that, I just know it in a lot of ways. The baby and I seemed to understand about that.

As a result of our morning's work, Don was aware of how awed he was by pregnancy and birth:

You know, no matter what we say about men and women and their individual part in producing a child, I am constantly awed by the wonder of it. Whatever you say about different societal attitudes towards birth over the centuries, giving birth is a power and a privilege. Something men are dwarfed by. . . . I never consider

that it's convenient for my wife to carry and bear our
child, that it's wonderful and that I don't have that
burden. I don't feel it's a burden at all. It's a mysterious
process . . . maybe that's why I unconsciously step back
from it because it's awesome and fearsome . . .
primordial. Maybe that's why I stare so much . . . as if
you are the goddess, the Divine Mother. . . .

His wife, Amy, found his reverent stares disconcerting; rather
than feeling admired, she felt his gaze to be distancing and impersonal. "I feel too earthy and needy to be larger than life."
    Other men also had a tendency to focus on the mythic aspects
of motherhood:

I thought about being born myself and about how we
feel we all share that primal attachment to the mother. I
felt identified with my baby and myself as baby and got
to feeling quite sentimental about my own mother as
goddess. Ye Gods, I've never thought of her in those
terms before.

One man picked up on the contrast between men's and
women's roles in childbearing:

Leni, I hear you suggesting that men envy women's
ability to carry a child in their bodies. I don't feel that
way at all. I feel I put the child there and I will have all
the benefits of having a child without the burden of
having to carry it around. So instead of feeling envy for
her ability to make a child grow, I feel quite the
opposite.

The group was momentarily silenced by the chauvinism of
that remark.
    The meditation was powerful for Rachel and Alan, who had

not yet conceived. Full of anxiety and questions about pregnancy and birth and parenthood, they felt delighted to be part of the group in order to eliminate emotional barriers to a possible conception.

> **Rachel**: Birth looms as such an overwhelming
> experience for me, I feel I might be swept away. The
> idea of the possible pain of labor and delivery terrifies
> me. I can't get past those spectres.

Before she met Alan, she'd had an abortion. Her guilt about that decision was still with her. During the morning exercise, her unresolved feelings about the abortion had been stirred up. Now, as she began to tell us the story, tears flooded down her face.

In talking about it with the group, Alan realized that it had remained. Each of us was caught up in our own emotional response as we listened. Alan recalled the time when she had first told him about her abortion. It remained a highly charged issue between them, especially now during their unsuccessful attempts to conceive. The trust level in the group deepened as Rachel risked her vulnerable feelings so openly. Silence followed. A comfortable pregnant silence.

The group was getting used to each other. Amy talked about the abortion she'd had some years before. It had been very scary and badly handled by the clinic, so she had strong empathy for Rachel. She went on to say that the memory was pretty dim now.

> I feel that's well behind me now. I was in touch with a
> sense of inadequacy when I was focusing on the exercise.
> I kept hearing myself say, "I'm still a kid, how can I be
> having a kid?" I hoped the baby wasn't listening.

Other reactions were voiced. Diverse feelings had been triggered by the exercise. Again and again in later sessions, I felt that the exercises were invaluable aids to bringing painful, repressed memories to the surface where they could be gently examined and correlated with present difficulties. Most often I didn't set a theme for any evening's discussion, and allowed the needs or mood of the group to determine what we dealt with on any given evening. Exercises that I had designed to help couples work on different issues were modified in the process of doing them to fit the moment. Often, highly volatile issues could best be dealt with by first participating in a group exercise in which no one was required to be analytical or rational about the concerns that were more often welling up from deep-seated emotional and subconscious levels.

Feelings of anger, frustration, confusion—a whole spectrum of heightened sensitivities, awakened by the stress of the transitional period, arose and needed to be examined in a supportive environment. Old childhood fantasies, anxieties and archetypal images that normally lay dormant in the subconscious rose to the surface of their everyday reality to trigger and unleash a whole Pandora's box of fears: fear of loss of control, of the unknown, dependency, rejection, incompetence—of death; death of one's self, of one's partner-provider, or the baby. It was clear that these themes did not arise only as discrete ideas, but were intertwined and interdependent themselves. Some themes were more resonant for one couple than another. For example, if, in one situation, a man did not give a woman enough appreciation for her developing pregnant body, she might tumble into despair. Another woman might not have any reaction. Old, lifelong patterns of acknowledgment—or lack of it—might be at the base of these responses.

One of the personal tasks assigned to group members was learning about their own biological births, about the circumstances and attitudes of their parents—whatever might throw light on conflicted and possibly even negative feelings about birth. The group, I felt, was a place in which experiences, possibly as traumatic as my own recollections which I had already shared with them, might be discussed in a supportive and explorative atmosphere.

As we met for three or four hours once a week over the months, couples relaxed, and in most cases, began to develop a new level of intimacy with each other and the group. As the sessions progressed during succeeding evenings, certain themes emerged in the group. Similar patterns were apparent in the groups that followed. The material that follows here is collected from about sixteen couples, although a typical group consisted of about five couples.

In later sessions, eating together seemed to be less important, for it appeared that the period of sociability diffused the feeling that had been incubating during the intervening week.

Instead of a meal together, I usually started the evening with a meditation or relaxation exercise to allow everyone to come together and to let go of the day's activities. This might be followed by another exercise which would catalyze feelings and help us to move to a deeper subjective level.

In the course of the workshops, we untangled many knotted strands of personal history which allowed a new self—a parent self—to evolve. Sometimes this happened through sudden "Ah, Ha!" insights, sometimes simply through the subtle realization that a certain stimulus no longer evoked a particular response. It seems to be true that one never quite knows how personal change takes place.

So much was going on all the time that it was hard to keep track of all the changes. We moved along, swept forward by the forceful physiological changes the women were undergoing. While we were actually meeting, I didn't categorize or label our discussions, but in retrospect it's clear that the classical themes of pregnancy arose again and again.

Ambivalence was a key issue early in everyone's pregnancy. Its intensity disappeared as the baby's actual presence became more apparent. Sometimes those ambivalent feelings reemerged in the eighth month as the baby's arrival became imminent.

At the beginning when the bulge was not yet apparent, pregnancy could either be kept a secret or announced with pride to all the world. Women dealt with it in quite different ways. Some preferred to become accustomed to the idea gradually, privately, slowly acknowledging the enormity of what was taking place deep within them. Often it was almost impossible to accept the reality of it all; as Elena put it:

* * *

What surprised me was the intensity of the revulsion I
occasionally felt when I considered the appearance of the
fetus in books like Nilsson's *A Child Is Born*. I really
didn't like the realization that *that* was inside me and
moving about.

Even women who were motivated toward pregnancy enter-
tained second thoughts. Often, eager to conceive, they still struggled against negative feelings during those first difficult weeks.
And then, after an initial adjustment, pregnancy seemed quite
natural and other matters quickly claimed their attention. After
her initial reluctance, Elena began to respond to the life force
within her. "It is like a tree that emerged from the ground and
needed to be nourished."

Adjusting to the reality of the pregnancy and its future implications is a subtle and continuing task for both mother and father.
Each has his own problems with it. On one occasion, I asked the
group whether this was a *planned* pregnancy and about their
reaction when they learned the news; there was an embarrassed
silence followed by nervous laughter.

Amy's reactions to her pregnancy were mixed. As a weaver,
who had only recently quit her job to weave full-time, she was
troubled by the ambivalence she felt and concerned that her
unresolved emotions might harm the child.

I was a little glad and a little sad. First of all I couldn't
believe it. I was over thirty and had never conceived. All
my friends had been having abortions for years. This is
the first year of my life when I'm doing what I want to
be doing and although Don is very sympathetic and I
really want to have this baby, I'm resenting it, too.

It was a relief, she said, to admit it out loud.
One man admitted he hadn't been ready for fatherhood at
all.

* * *

I seriously considered an abortion for us, but now that I
see my wife's belly, I realize it was outrageous.

Elena: Planned? It's hard to say . . . right now my
fantasies are pretty scary sometimes. Whenever I'm
feeling fearful or worried about what it's going to be like
to be a mother or even whether I really want it, I start
to feel guilty. That's when I imagine that the baby wants
to get even with me. . . . I feel it knows what I'm
thinking

Anne: I can't believe it's really happening to
me . . . that I'm pregnant, that we're going to have a
child. Sam's delighted, I'm scared. It's a relief to know
others have fears, too, that it happens with other
people . . . that it's O.K. to have fears. Maybe I can
begin to share some of the warm pleasurable feelings,
too.

Ria and Eric's story leaked out gradually and was never fully
revealed until after the baby was born, when Eric revealed to me
that he'd been extremely ambivalent early in the pregnancy but
afraid to reveal it. Ria, on the other hand, dealt with issues more
openly during the group:

Yesterday I went to visit a friend who has a six-year-old,
a three-year-old and a four-month-old baby. It was great
to hold the baby, I think that's why I headed for her
house. I was also overwhelmed by the horrible sense of
what it means to bring into one's house a little creature
who can never again be left alone and is such an
enormous and inescapable responsibility. I realized that
I have chosen such a responsibility, and that I don't

know what I have gotten myself and Eric into. . . . I guess I feel a little more peaceful about all that but it isn't resolved yet.

Only much later, long after the births, when I asked people to reflect on their experiences in the group, did I discover the intensity of the feelings involved for Eric and Ria.

Often it was through journals kept during the workshops that people were able to express conflicts and emotional turmoil. Sometimes entries were read out loud. Usually, it was the women who wrote. Anne had started keeping a journal even before joining the group.

I feel trapped. Maybe an abortion. It's not happening to me. It's a movie and I'll play a part (simpering motherhood, cherubic smile) but I don't feel it. I'm numb. Next, I'm scared. What have we done? Dreams of death—my dear parents' deaths. One night, stark terror, nameless.

I haven't been able to completely shake that terror that I felt that night six-eight weeks ago, when I woke up in the middle of the night absolutely terrified in the depths of my being . . . pure terror, unlike anything I'd ever felt except maybe as a young child. Nothing Sam or anyone else could do could reach it. It reaches to the core of me.

Oh my God, there's nothing I can do, nothing you can do, nothing to be done. It's finally happening, it's happened. A baby! The dread—maybe it will happen—is replaced by certainty. Oh God, Oh Lord, there's nothing we can do, I can do.

Occasionally, I have little episodes of fear, rising from the solar plexus through chest to throat where I succeed in choking it off. Like when I heard Hal describing the research on care of infants just after birth. I don't want to hear about it. Or like when I am

telling people I am pregnant. The same rising wave.
Some of the fear escapes from my eyes.

And then after the first couple of sessions:

Sometimes I feel smug. I'll be sitting in a meeting at
work and think, there's something very special
happening and you all don't know what it's like.

Her later entries showed steady progress in accepting the
pregnancy:

At Christmas, I pop out, begin to show. I start telling
friends and office mates—a great relief not to have some
secret, almost like a malignant disease! I relax more. The
Cleopatra idea fits in here, I begin to let the positive
feelings well up. Still some uncertainty but I'm getting
grounded.
   Lately, I've been asking myself why can't I take this
motherhood thing in stride? Why does it seem so earth
shattering? I'm going to be more mature, take it in
stride. Feeling anxious and expressing it can be
overdone. . . . I haven't expressed my competent side
enough.
   Sam is really delighted about the offspring (his
drawing of skipping father with big heart which he drew
in the group). . . . He doesn't show this very directly in
the group; he stays at a philosophic conceptual level
most of the time—but then seeing him in the group
allows me to see that these joyful feelings are there for
him, too. The nonverbal work helps our sharing. Sam's
and mine.

We noticed symptoms of pregnancy such as nausea, swelling
bellies and food cravings among some of the men in the group—

classical *couvade* symptoms. One man had back pain for four months, beginning in the fifth month of his wife's pregnancy. He noted in his journal:

> I thought I was going to be wheeled into the delivery room with Nancy. I joked about the serious pain in my back; it was so embarrassing. It seemed obvious it was connected to the baby. It struck me that it was like hiccoughing for two days straight before our wedding.

Another man told us that at his birth, his father developed shingles right afterwards. This meant that his mother and he had to remain in the hospital until a nurse could be found to take care of all of them at home.

Many fathers in the group were awed by the developing pregnancy and felt distant from the experience. Some were able to acknowledge that they felt envious of their wives' biological role.

> **Dick:** Sure, I'm jealous. Sure, I would like to carry a baby. It must be colossal of course, there is the weight and the discomfort, but to feel this thing growing inside of me!

> **Alan:** Men go around biologically unfulfilled in a way. Perhaps there is envy of the satisfaction that comes with completing certain biological life cycles. How many life cycles do men complete . . . just birth and death? Somehow ejaculation is not the same thing. I envy the stress a woman feels as she passes through the big event.

> **Eric:** I was never consciously envious, though I have some friends who have gone through giving birth trips— pseudodeliveries and pseudobirths. . . .
> I don't feel as if I had much responsibility in the creation of the baby. It's a little weird to me, but then I say to myself . . . who else is responsible?

* * *

In the midst of one such discussion, I suggested that it would be more effective if the men really tried to imagine what it would be like to be pregnant rather than talking about it so abstractly. We decided to perform the exercise called "Father's Fantasy of Being Pregnant." I asked them to stuff pillows under their shirts and sit in a circle in the middle of the room. The wives were delighted. After a moment or two of silence, I began to guide them into a fantasy of pregnancy. They sat with eyes closed, sensing their expanded shape, swollen with the life inside it.

Close your eyes. Breathe gently and naturally, allowing
your breath to rise and fall without changing its rhythm.
Feel your belly with your hands. Feel the roundness of
it, the firmness of it, feel the pressure of the uterus
against your chest and the bulge resting on your lap.
Your belly has been growing gradually for the past
months—you are seven months pregnant. You are
feeling full and ripe. The baby is moving about inside
you, kicking, turning, making its presence felt.

I asked them to speak when they felt the urge. It didn't take long for the words to come.

It's like having a nice companion with me, but I don't
like having a big belly; it's getting in my way. It keeps
me away from other people. I have a feeling of
disfigurement. At first I just felt I had a pillow against
my stomach and I felt silly, but then I thought what if I
had to watch it grow slowly. I imagine I might feel some
resentment about it. It's a tumor; I'm glad I can take the
pillow out and put the whole thing away. I'm just as
happy to let someone else carry it. How's yours?

* * *

Dick: Great! We "women" are lucky. It allows us to keep in touch with the cosmos. I think my belly is a majestic thing, a fantastic thing. It is like a drum, this taut thing, full of life. I'm proud of this bulging belly, not at all disfigured. What's disfiguring? It's life!

After the exercise, Amy spoke:

I've always been glad to be on this side of it and felt sorry for men. I always wondered how they felt, so I'm relieved that they don't feel that they are missing a lot. Now I can be greedy about enjoying my pregnant state.

Leni: And might you want to go one step further and tell Don what you would like over and beyond being able to enjoy this state or what might help you get even more out of it?

Amy: I want you to appreciate me as a woman and really feel the life and the movement inside me all the time. . . . It never seems to stop. I want you to feel the wonder of it the way I do and the beauty . . . and the beauty of my form, too. I want you to feel part of the whole thing. I want you to say to people . . . "Look, that's my wife and my kid."

Although most of the women loved their changing form, their productive interior, it brought with it continuing problems of self-image and feelings of intrusion. Early in the pregnancy, before the baby's movements were felt, Amy was sorting out the "I feel the bulge is me and yet not me" feelings. Later on, as Amy's form swelled, the pregnancy was undeniable, yet still hard to fully absorb on a deeper psychological level:

Who am I in relation to this intruder who is taking over my body? It is a problem for me: I wake up in the night feeling outraged at this insistent being, this parasitic intruder inside my body.

Anne wrote in her journal during the first months:

The knowing, from the first weeks, of the change, of the activity and the *presence*, especially the presence. No longer a space but a form, an energy.
    Knowing, but at first not wanting to believe. And yet, hiding a Mona Lisa smile. . . .
    I've touched the edge of time and space. I'm connected to it, the link is made.

Ria: I caught a glimpse of myself in the mirror—the full-length mirror in the locker room at the pool at school—and I pulled my dress in to outline my belly. I still can't believe it's a baby, that I'm really pregnant as I've imagined being, as I've hoped I'd be, almost all my life.

Jean: My father-in-law and I have bellies that meet, but he doesn't like me to point it out. The funniest thing about my changing shape is growing so big that I can't even see my feet when I look down. Since I know it's temporary, I play games about being a fat person and having a big belly.

Many were proud of their changing form and the new status it implied, and longed for everyone to notice.

Elena: I feel I'm very beautiful to myself and Dick. I'm doting on that. I love my developing belly.

Some women worried about losing their appeal. An animated

discussion developed around that issue one night. Feelings tumbled out.

Elena: When a pregnant friend and I walk together on the street and catch sight of our roly-poly reflections in the store windows, we go into gales of laughter like adolescents. But if our husbands laugh at our misshapen bodies, or our transient moods, it's another matter. We get quite depressed.

Amy: I was thinking that you never see a pregnant pin-up. I've been looking at a lot of birth books—some of the pictures are so striking—the beauty and sensuality of the roundness. Sometimes when I shower, I just look at this big belly and love that it is there.

Elena persisted quietly:

But sometimes I feel quite fat and ugly and I find myself watching other women's bodies. Do you have that problem? I find I go into a tailspin, afraid that Dick will stray away.

This is the first time in my life that I've had some physical limitation and, of course, I realize it is indicative of the whole change of life-style.

Self-image, dependency, trust were all inextricably entangled in this transition from being a couple to becoming a family. These strands were woven through the workshop.

Beth: After the struggle to be independent and autonomous, I was suddenly so vulnerable and dependent in every conceivable way. Fortunately, it never came out in resentment towards the baby.

* * *

In response to Beth's increasing and uncharacteristic neediness, Nick admitted he often found himself withholding the very affection and nurturing that she needed to feel comforted or turned-on sexually. When this happened, they would retire to their corners in a tangle of confusion and misunderstanding. Both would end up suffering.

There were repetitive themes underlying the conflicts that arose between partners:

- Are you hearing me?
- Will you respond to me?
- Can I depend on you?
- Can I trust you?

For many men, it became difficult to handle the increased demands and dependency, threatened as they were by their own feelings of insecurity in anticipation of a third person in their lives. In the groups, they were encouraged to examine tensions as they arose, rather than withdrawing or keeping up a good front.

One week Elena and Dick arrived, furious at each other. Most of the evening was devoted to clarifying what had happened to them since the last session of the group. It had started over a simple thing. Elena had wanted Dick to go to a meeting with her one night. He said no. She took it as a personal rejection. It became a matter of his inattention.

The following week Elena came back, looking radiant.

It was so good to be able to work that problem out here. I think it was getting it out in a situation that was safe, with people who had similar concerns . . . that's been really helpful, because I felt good this week and I felt that Dick and I were good together this week. If we had a similar discussion at home it would have just . . . in fact, we have had similar discussions, and it didn't clarify anything. I don't think we always need people, but I think on that sticky issue we worked through, it was really helpful.

Misunderstandings related to increased dependency were a major problem for most couples. Sometimes the conflict went like this:

Alan: Reconnecting at the end of the day is a problem. When I come home, Rachel's been home all day; she wants to share her experience of the day—but even though I've come home, I'm still working—I want to complete some telephone calls, make some notes. . . . She wants to connect and I'm experiencing something else. I really feel pushed.

Rachel: Sure you answer me, but I need something more from you—a reaction, for instance—I imagine something is going on in you, you're upset and not sharing it and I hesitate to say other things and it starts a whole spiral of angry behavior and missed signals.

Often, conflicts reflect patterns of unresolved behavior from childhood and the pregnant period becomes a time to confront it once again and work it through, often with more satisfying, conclusive results. I suggested that evening that Rachel and Alan try a Gestalt exercise called "I Resent." They were asked to sit opposite each other and trade resentments. Alan began.

I resent it when you involve me the moment I walk in the door. I resent it when you want me to listen to the events of your day whether they were positive or a drag. . . .

* * *

After a mechanical start, Alan warmed to the task; he poured out a long list of resentments, becoming more and more emotional as he progressed. Rachel was instructed to sit quietly and listen without responding. She then followed with her list of past and present grievances and resentments. Rachel expressed surprise at how familiar the resentments sounded, commenting, "I sound like my mother, for God's sake." It was a catharsis, to be sure, and also an opportunity to observe how one can project childhood resentments onto present circumstances.

> **Alan:** It sure is something to guard against in the future. I realize that if Rachel gives me space to unwind and get my head clear and then I still don't come around, or respond after a while, she sure has a valid complaint. I really have to acknowledge that negative behavior, then.

After they finished exchanging resentments, they spent a little time with the positive side of the same exercise called "I Appreciate," which worked in a similar fashion. At the end of the exercise, they discussed how they might spend time together at the end of the work day, when each needed contact but might not be ready to talk. For instance, they considered as a homecoming ritual taking a bath together, massaging each other, or just lying quietly on the bed in each other's arms—gentle ways to be in touch, ways to sense rather than using words to explain their mood. They talked of including the unborn baby in their new homecoming ritual, and were pleased that the exercise had worked so well. For them, as for many of us, words tend to be such a habitual way of connecting that we forget the power of a tender exchange expressed through touch, and the importance of gentling one another.

After Rachel and Alan had resolved their differences, the group participated in "Hand Conversation," a nonverbal communication exercise. Partners stood opposite each other and grasped hands as if in meeting. They were limited to expressing themselves through their hands: feelings of pleasure, anger, impatience, or whatever was present. Afterward, we discussed the emotions the exercise evoked. Some people had been surprised by the way the play had turned into aggression. Others found their connection very sensual.

The next week, Rachel reported that the "I Resent" exercise had really helped her to see Alan's point of view. Rachel said thoughtfully:

> If I tackle Alan at the door with either my enthusiasm or my neediness, I hear my inner voice saying "You've done it again!"

For most men, it was difficult to accompany their partners on the emotional roller coaster of pregnancy, since their hormones weren't providing them with the same momentum.

> **Don:** It's not only that Amy's normal emotions are amplified, but I simply tune in to a different channel in life.
> Yes, I guess, I tune out because I feel so inadequate. I don't know how to even begin to be comforting, since I don't have any familiarity with such highs and lows.

Lovemaking, a form of intense, tender communication that might normally dissipate some of this distance, can itself become a source of misunderstanding and hurt feelings during pregnancy.

Some women in the groups became withdrawn, self-absorbed and turned-off sexually as the pregnancy advanced. Others felt passive and more dependent. They needed affection and cuddling more than sex. Jan, at eight months, said:

> I feel disinterested in sex but I'm worried about being

indifferent and turned off. I'm afraid Peter will wander off and have an affair.

Elena had similar feelings:

We need each other but in different ways. For instance, I want to be held and cuddled and Dick wants to have intercourse. It causes a lot of tension when we can't talk it through.

Ironically, whether women wanted less sex or more sex, they worried about their partners' responses to their new patterns. As one might expect, many women experienced a heightened interest during the early months, and often felt anxious about making too many demands on their husbands. Others felt confused by the simultaneous, competitive pull between the roles of wife, lover and mother. There was a continuing problem of learning to talk clearly about intensified needs and fears:

Alan: Underneath the disagreeableness we get into, is the question, "Why aren't you there for me?" followed by "Is this what's going to happen in the future?" It's the fear of that.

Rachel: I'm thinking the same thing . . . "Am I going to be left with the kid all the time?"

Anne: We still have problems asking for what we need but we're getting better. Practicing here in the group helps. I seem to be asking for more, at least that's what Sam says, although I feel I'm still asking for the same old things—to be seen and heard. Maybe, the volume is just turned up now—Our professional lives have been quite separate. We have had different orbits for a long time, but now the pregnancy is bringing us more together, and I think the baby will do that even more.

Rachel: Why is a demand automatically a big awkward thing?

Alan: It is as if at times I am treated without personal respect, as though things were expected of me. I have to do it, it doesn't matter if I do it out of love or not, it just is expected.

In the groups, we found people had a safe place where they could risk being vulnerable in order to open up communication with their partners.

Beth: I've had a hard time this week and I realize I don't know how to ask Nick for help for my little-girl self. I don't know whether I'm asking for it for my wife-grown-up self or for my little-girl self. I want to say, "Please, Nick, protect me. I need you."

It's important that you let this little girl that's in me get protection because I never got if from my father . . . at least a sense of physical stroking and protection. My father never held me, he never stroked me, he never kissed me and said, "Don't worry." When Nick gives me that, I feel that I can go on. . . .

Leni: Have you ever told him that directly?

Beth: I think I have.

Leni: Try telling him that directly, because I noticed that you were just addressing your remarks to all of the rest of us.

Beth: There is a big part of me that needs a father and needs everything a father can give: attention, love, affection. I have needed to know that a father would soothe my crying and make me feel good again. You are giving that to me and it really fills me up.

Nick: That really makes me feel good.

Leni: Did you know that?

Nick: I know I was trying. I didn't know I was successful.

The men's needs for sex and affection varied as much as the women's. Some felt aroused by their partners' developing bodies. Others felt disinterested, timid or even repelled, expressing their discomfort by withdrawing and becoming emotionally inaccessible or unconsciously spending more time away from home. As their partners became more introverted and passive through the months, the subsequent loss of attention sometimes became equated with loss of love.

Nick: When Beth is so self-absorbed, I feel slighted by the lack of attention, and I find myself becoming interested in other women. I feel like a heel.

In the first week, Dick wrote in his journal:

I feel apart with you, farther than we have been in months, sometimes so far that it's as if I don't know you. I miss you. You're sleeping a lot and lying around a lot. A feeling of a friend rejected comes across me, but I don't reject you, too. Perhaps I could massage you; I don't. I walk the dog for you, buy specially requested food for you, cook for myself and eat alone. Isn't that enough? Must I make love to you, too? You are a beautiful woman and increasingly so. But are you still the sexy woman? Seducing me and wanting me between your legs like you did a month ago? Prove it. You must come to me, not I to you.

Another father felt responsible for "ruining" his wife's body, as it became more and more "distended." One admitted that his image of his wife's breasts changed from a source of erotic pleasure to an image of two hanging milk dispensers. Such admissions were not easy to make, but helped clear the way for better interactions. A few couples, however, had an active sex life until the last day, making love hours before labor started—despite their doctor's admonitions.

Nancy: A great need came over me to be with John, but he was so immersed in his work that he didn't even seem to be aware of me. I started picking a fight with him, which was my sneaky way of getting him to pay attention to me. I started sobbing . . . I thought he didn't care. Of course, that wasn't true. He took me home and we made love. I knew instinctively that labor would not be far away after it. I think that was what my need was, to attend to myself pregnant, in the last hours of fullness, rather than let them slip away unacknowledged. At three A.M. I awoke John because I felt the birth waters oozing.

Dick was one of those who enjoyed each new development of his partner's changing body and felt aroused by her pregnant state:

I feel no less lust for her now than I ever did. In fact, I feel more attracted to her. It's simply one more aspect of the woman I love.

Beth felt beautiful and sexy, up until the last week:

I'm doting on it—and my feeling of sexuality has been heightened. But in the past month (the ninth) I don't feel like having sex because I'm so puffy—orgasm is no longer down there, it feels like branches all around my body.

* * *

Ria wrote in her journal:

> I feel progressively less need for sexual intercourse as the
> pregnancy progresses, but increasing need for other
> physical contact with Eric—expressions of affection,
> concern, protection. More than sex.

Toward the end of pregnancy, it was a relief to be able to share problems about sex openly, knowing others in the group would understand.

> **Jean:** The lack of sexuality worried me. I didn't want
> sex, but I was worried that he didn't either. That was
> risky and scary. We got into a whole thing about who
> initiates sex. We couldn't even fit our bodies into each
> other. It was absurd—we had a few tragic episodes—I'd
> get a cramp—he'd freak and say, "It's moving"—it was
> hopeless.
>
> **Beth:** I know Nick felt he was hurting me or sometimes
> the baby and I felt awful about my body. It never
> worked by the end. And yet we really needed each other
> in that intimate way.

As developing bellies and the baby's movements confirmed the reality of the pregnancy, concern over impending motherhood became intertwined with thoughts of one's own mother. In the fourth and fifth months, women in the group began to relate to their mothers and the whole world of women in ways they hadn't for years. They were realizing that they were going to be mothers as well as daughters, just as their mothers were before them. Ria, whose mother lived in far distant Wisconsin, told us:

> I've been having a lot of feelings about my mother

recently, angry feelings—wanting my mother to be more of what she isn't—more available on a deeper level. My mother is never available and I have been feeling a lot of resentment about that recently. Underneath is the fear that I will be that kind of mother, too. I want to be more giving and to be given to.

Elena: Actually, I'm finding that my relationship with my mother isn't changed really, but there are subtle differences, especially in my attitude toward her. I feel more in need of her and I think of her frequently and feel more admiring of her now more than ever.

When I had morning sickness, there were a couple of times when I just thought, "I want my mother." I felt as sick as I ever did when I was a kid and I want the total attention my mother gave where every need was answered.

Anne was sitting next to her, crosslegged on the floor, supporting her back against Sam's legs. Leaning over to Elena, she touched her hand and quipped:

I really know that feeling but I realized that I don't want *my* mother. I want an archetypical one, the *perfect* mother, don't you?

In their second trimester, women in the groups typically moved from a concern for their relationship with their mothers, to a preoccupation with their relationship to their partners. Most of the women in the groups expressed an increasing need for their husband's affection and concern. Often, they felt quite dependent and needed reassurance, beyond what they themselves felt was acceptable or rational. By now the baby had "quickened in the womb," its activity a constant affirmation that it was alive and well; nevertheless, the women would often fret about whether things were progressing normally. Most of the men found these obsessive concerns difficult to deal with.

Peter: I struggled to meet Jan's emotional needs, but often it got the best of me and I feel quite inadequate. After a while, I felt drained. No matter what I did, it was never enough. I began to feel hopeless. There was only so much attention I could give Jan—only so much hand-holding and reassurance. In a tribal society, there are more people around to help tend to the women.

Eric: How many times can I assure Ria that the baby is not going to be a monster? I get very impatient.

They worried about what would happen in the future, after the baby arrived.

Elena: I'm afraid it's going to be me and the baby together and Dick by himself out there. I get frightened and then he gets angry and then I get angry and I feel responsible, I want Dick to feel responsible, too. I want to know that I'm not in this alone.

They wanted their partner's involvement and sharing.

Anne: I want you to feel the wonder of it just the way I feel the wonder of this unknown being who is soon to be known to us. I want you to know how it feels when the baby touches me inside. . . .

Don: With the most sympathetic interest and involvement, it is still something that is not happening to us—during the pregnancy, I'm a spectator.

Dick: It's the most exceptional, and at the same time,

routine miracle in the world—a woman is just doing
what she's meant to do normally. Of course, I realize it's
not routine to Elena, just collectively.

Don: Whatever you say about different societal attitudes
over the centuries, giving birth is a power and a
privilege—something that men are dwarfed by. I think it
is a mysterious thing—maybe that is why I take a step
back from it, it is awesome and fearful.

But Amy wanted to be *human*:

I don't want to be looked at like some goddess figure. I
want your attention to be personal.

Men, too, were moving through a similar transformation as
they became fathers to their children instead of sons to their
fathers. Historically, men have been fearful of the transformative
power of birth and in many cultures the birth process is placed in
a dangerous category. Some of that carries over for both men and
women now. In the groups, men and women alike harbored
uncomfortable feelings about the messiness, bloodiness and
potential danger of birth, remarking that they had read and heard
it was a violent experience. One evening we spent time free-
associating, starting with words such as blood, sex, mother, birth,
breasts, pain, etc. Surprisingly negative attitudes and feelings
were expressed.

Peter: When I think of birth, I can only think of all
that stuff coming out . . . and of how bloody and
dangerous it is.

Or women thought more specifically about the baby when they
thought of birth.

* * *

I am worried about whether the baby will be normal. I was reading the *Time-Life* book on birth today, which is such an inhumane book, although an informational book, but saying things like—one of the most amazing things is that almost all of the systems in the baby have to start working right away . . . for instance, the lungs have never worked before. What if the lungs don't work, and the heart has only worked in a very simple way, and something new happens to the circulatory system when the baby's born. It changes, and what if it doesn't work?

Loss of control over one's body and over one's future became an imminent reality toward the end.

Jean: The loss of control over what happens inside me is apparent when I lie down to go to sleep. When I want to sleep, the baby starts to kick and I want to scream, "Stop!" I feel as if I am being taken over and things are moving much too fast. And that, quite possibly, I'm afraid to go to sleep for fear that I'll discover by morning that the baby has taken flight.

Thoughts of death were common toward the end. There was an intuitive sense that one's old self had to die, to be relinquished in order for the new parent self to born. But it was a struggle to accept the necessity of this transformation. One night, Ria confided:

I have a fear of losing self—it's like a death—withering away and ecstasy are both a losing of self and I am fearful of both—of being carried away. Perhaps it is possible to go with the feelings no matter what they are.

Anne: It's a point of vulnerability in your life, physical vulnerability. There's so much that's essential about life that's going on, but death is also present. I've become aware of both of them at the same time.

Although we talked about problems that might arise during labor and throughout the four months, as the time of birth neared for some of the first couples, we focused more directly on specific questions and feelings. Fears were voiced about losing control, about one's ability to deal with pain, about trusting others to be there, giving support—fears about the unknown experience ahead.

And perhaps, underlying the unknown and the unpredictable aspects was the known—the unconscious "memory" for both parents of their own biological births, as Grof's and Sagan's theories suggest—colored by the fragments of recollections that parents hand down to all of us. These half-remembered memories and stories may make us wary of reexperiencing the birth trauma once again, through the birth of our own children. There may also be an unconscious resistance to causing one's own baby pain during birth.

These kinds of fears can, indeed, affect the course of labor. Emotional anxiety can cause delays in contractions or create tension in uterine muscles, resulting in increased pain and prolongation of labor. As fear persists, the body responds by drawing blood away from the uterus toward organs of defense. As a result, the baby moving out of the womb and into the birth canal is deprived of the oxygenated blood on which its life depends, until it can start breathing on its own. Therefore it is of utmost importance to the well-being of both mother and child to give the kind of support that will dispel fear. Although this may seem obvious now, it is essential to understand the biological consequences of anxiety, so that it can be eliminated as an inevitable aspect of childbearing. The best way to provide the needed support will be different for each mother.

In the early 1970s group members had few alternatives to

traditional hospital delivery in the New York area. Along with the majority of the population of the United States, cultural attitudes influenced their choice in favor of delivering in the hospital. Just like their parents, they followed the convention of the day. Decades before that, it was natural for their grandmothers to give birth at home in their own beds, attended by family physician or midwife, surrounded by their families. But, at this time, for these couples, the safety of the hospital environment, the modern technology of the delivery room and the care of the medical specialist were all crucial. So, all chose an obstetrician and planned to deliver in the hospital with which the doctor was affiliated. All couples attended a six-week "prepared" childbirth class that taught them techniques to make labor easier. I encouraged them to do this, because I felt that, if possible, giving birth with a minimum of drugs was preferable for the well-being of baby and mother. In the group, therefore, rather than concentrating on preparing for alternative ways of giving birth, we worked on the underlying feelings and emotions that *any* labor and delivery process would evoke.

Different couples had very different worries about issues concerning the medical aspects of birth. On one evening near the end of the group, the recurrent issue of trust arose. This time it centered on the doubts Elena and Beth began to feel about their doctors.

Elena: Since this is my first birth, I feel I have a right to go to Dr. F. with my questions, even my simple questions, let alone the ones that I sense but can't articulate yet.

You see, although I knew I could get answers to my questions out of a book, I wanted them from my doctor. I wanted his respect; I wanted him to know I could ask intelligent questions, that I knew what it was about. Because up until now, I've been sort of mute, which seems to be agreeable with him. . . . I mean, he would say, "Do you have any questions?" and while saying that be jumping out of the chair on the way to seeing the next person. So his attitude wasn't very conducive to an open exchange. It's as if I'm trying to say I want you to *see* me.

Beth: I used to make a list of questions to ask my doctor, and, with my heart pounding for fear he'd refuse to answer, rush them all out, as he backed out the door. Often, about a symptom, he'd say, "That's normal," leaving me totally dependent on his reassurance, without any information to help me be able to reassure myself.

We used another role-playing exercise in which Elena played the role of the doctor and others in the group played the roles of patient and husband. We acted out the office visit, asking all the questions that Elena was finding most difficult to articulate or even remember in the rushed exchange. As she took the role of her doctor, it allowed her to understand the doctor's position more clearly, and as her behavior was mirrored by someone else playing her part, it helped her to see her part in the interaction. We rehearsed the visit several times, finding that repetition brought self-confidence.

Many women in the group shared the fear that the doctor wouldn't be there with the emotional support they needed during labor. Hearing some of their friends' experiences had reinforced their anxiety and distrust. They also worried that they might lose courage at the last minute during labor and, despite their "training" and resolve to give birth without drugs, they might "chicken out."

One evening a casual discussion about the merits of home delivery resulted in an animated discussion involving trust of doctors and hospitals. Everyone interrupted each other in a rush to express themselves. It was a hot issue. We talked about control and about fear of the loss of control, and about taking responsibility for how we wanted things to happen. The men expressed confidence in the technological backup systems that would be available in the hospital environment. In contrast, many of the women not only were totally untrusting of this technology, but felt deeply threatened by the possibility of induced labor, fetal monitors, drugged delivery—all of it. Don had started out calmly and rationally:

> I feel that the doctor is a professional: he knows what he's about, he's had a lot of training to do this and I trust him. I like to go to doctors.

But his partner, Amy, disagreed passionately:

> I resent doctors and hospitals. I feel as if I am putting myself in somebody else's hands. They don't tell you what they are doing and that includes my own doctor. I feel they are going to do something *to* me and not tell me. . . . They are going to take it out of my hands at the hospital. That's been my experience everytime I'm involved with a doctor.

Anne: I feel the same way really strongly.

Amy: I've been carrying this baby for nine months—it's been eating with me, living with me. . . . By God, I've brought it this far, I can carry it the rest of the way.

Ria: Aren't you partly responsible for the way that happens? Can't you say to your doctor, "I don't want anything to happen to me without being specifically told"?

Anne: You can say that but some resident can come along and he's ready to induce and zap. . . .

Amy: You bet. The doctor gives me pat answers; he never explains anything no matter what I ask him. I see Don's role as fighting the doctor because I'm not going to have time to fight the doctor.

Eric: Can I ask you a question? Why in the world do you go to that doctor?

Amy: Because he's a good doctor.

Eric: Bullshit!

The evening ended with the issue unresolved, but the following week, we acted out a fantasy exercise in which we rehearsed the birth.

In another group, it was Ruth who was close to term, who began to worry about the feasibility of carrying out their plans.

> **Ruth:** Though I'm planning to have natural childbirth, I'm scared I might get scared at the end. I'll need my doctor's support then and where will he be? I want to be sure he'll be there as a guide and won't take it away from me at the last minute by making a decision *for* me, saying, "Oh, well, she's not doing too well, I'd better induce."

Like the others, Ruth was concerned about being pressured into accepting last-minute medical interventions, as had many of her friends.

At the next session, Ruth came to the workshop directly from her doctor's office, in a fury:

> I suddenly thought—who's in charge of all this? I am! Damn it. It's my body, my baby. It's hard to get into an accepting frame of mind when I ask the doctor questions and he answers, "This is the way we do it in the hospital. . . . It is in your best interest." I come away believing for a while. I begin to agree with his reasoning. Yes, I really need an I.V. because if something goes wrong I might need an operation (Does that become a self-fulfilling prophecy?), and I need an episiotomy because the tissue might rip and that would be terrible. . . . I need a monitor because the cord may

strangle the baby or it may be stillborn but with this
machine, they will save my baby. I begin to believe all
these horror stories—it introduces all my worst fears and
pretty soon I'm convinced. After all, I've gone to him
assuming he knows. It's hard to say no, but damn, I'm
yielding all my power to him—my mother instinct, the
thing I trust inside. Suddenly I say to myself, wait a
minute, I can't *trust* this doctor.

Ruth and her partner, Harvey, a psychiatrist at a large New
York medical center, were concerned about planning how they
wanted their birth to be and were afraid that hospital rules and
regulations would prevent them from carrying it out their way.
Since Harvey was a doctor, he had first-hand knowledge of the
system. Barring unforeseen complications, they wanted to design
it their way. Ultimately they did—although the outcome was not
what they had expected. In Chapter V: The First Group Gives
Birth, and in Chapter VI: Patterns and Reflections: The Group
Looks Back, their experience as well as that of others is described
in relation to their long preparation in the group.

V

The First Group Gives Birth

It was such a miracle that first there was just
one person, and suddenly there were two.

—Sara, thirty-three, after the birth of Michael

Several weeks after the first workshop series had formally ended, we gathered once again to tell our stories. Three out of five babies had been born, and two couples had brought their infants to show them off to the group. More importantly, we wanted to share the details of the birth experiences before the intensity of the memories was lost. Of course, there had been the euphoric telephone calls immediately after the births to all of us as "extended family," but this evening of minute detail was an important follow-up. We were delighted to see each other.

Hearing this information had significant ramifications for the parents of the babies who had not yet been born. The exchanges that evening dramatically altered how some decided to shape the environment of their birth experience.

Part of the ritual of becoming a mother is adding one's own history of giving birth to that of all the mothers who have given birth. It is not without meaning that thirty years later, a woman can tell her story in minute detail. Each mother is a central figure in the retelling of the mythic story of creation—the heroine's journey. It is akin to men telling their war stories—the hero's journey.

The relating of the birth story can become unexpectedly poetic, as in the following journal entry from Sara:

153

*   *   *

When the time came to push, a surge went rippling
through my body and soul demanding that I bear down
so that I could push life into the world like all the other
women before me who have chosen to be passage to life.
   Within seconds of his head crowning, his body
slipped out of mine, an ooze and a swish that felt
glorious and was too quickly gone. Like seeing the
morning sunrise, there are no words to speak my heart
at this moment. I am in awe. I ache.

As the women talked, I was aware of a fascinating change in the
group's interactions. This change was striking to me: after so
many months of intimacy, couples who had babies were now
absorbed in the demands of parenthood. These concerns had
catapulted them beyond the reach of their still-pregnant friends.
The latter were still coping with some of their fears about the
unknown and unpredictable transition that lay ahead of them.
There was an unacknowledgable, subtle emotional distance
between the two groups—those who had crossed the bridge into
the future and those who waited to do so. And the tiny members of
the group, who had been present but not seen before, became an
irresistible focus of attention, try as we might to cling to the old
group patterns. Gradually, the group molded itself to include
these wonderful new distractions. It was moving to see mothers
who had worried so about their competence caring for their babies
as if they had been doing so forever.
   Of the three births, two were complicated hospital deliveries
that had proved to be quite traumatic for the whole family.
   Even after attending a support group such as ours, and having
the advantage of more preparation than usual, parents had
remained powerless to carry out their plans. It was clear that the
medical system, even in these different "excellent" hospitals of
the parents' choice, was not responsive to the essence and nature
of the birth event. This revelation affected one still-expectant
couple so strongly that they began making plans for a home

delivery at a friend's house near their hospital. Ria and Eric, whose delivery was less stressful, were able to carry out their personal plans more successfully.

Amy and Don

Amy and Don's experience of labor and delivery was, they believed, not what they had expected—or wanted—at all.

It's amazing. It was nothing like anything I was prepared for beforehand. I remember feeling that with all my reading and all of my exercise and our work together here, I was going to have a snap of a time. Never did I consider that it would be as it was.

First of all, Amy's doctor was on vacation, so his partner took over. He sent her to the hospital when she was dilated three centimeters and in the course of the next eight hours, her labor moved along very slowly; she dilated only one more centimeter. Nurses and interns came and went as day staff were replaced by night staff.

As soon as I became comfortable with one, he or she turned into another. The doctor came in and told me he could speed up my labor by giving me Pitocin. I knew that meant it would be much more painful and they would have to give me painkilling drugs to offset the pain. I was not prepared for that. Never had I considered that I would take any kind of anesthesia because of its effect on the baby. When I asked him what was happening, he told me he didn't know but it must be something in my midbrain. I didn't know what happened in my midbrain, but I figured that it was

something psychological. I figured I wasn't natural
enough to have natural childbirth. I got very upset and
even more tense. He never even explained to me what
happens in your midbrain.

The doctor and nurses put pressure on Amy to agree to having
an epidural (spinal anesthetic). Don was enlisted to convince her,
too. They told her if she had an epidural and used Pitocin, she
would have the baby in three hours; otherwise her labor might
continue in the same slow, ineffective way for twelve hours.

Amy: I didn't know what to do as they kept saying, "It's
up to you. If I were you, I'd want to get it over with."

Reluctantly, feeling like a failure, she agreed.
As Amy talked that evening, I remembered something she'd
said during an earlier workshop session. She had expressed her
anxiety about submitting to the medical system, since a previous
experience in the hospital for a small operation had been a bad
one, in which they never told her what they were doing.

When they gave me the spinal, they hit a nerve. I was so
scared. I said, "Get away from me. Don't touch me. I'll
do this birth myself." "O.K.," they said, "if that's the
way you feel," and they took out everything and walked
out. The doctor got mad at me and wouldn't talk to me.
One thing led to another. Meanwhile, I was in a lot of
pain. Don was pressuring me to get them back in to
administer the spinal again. Hours passed, no further
dilation, no progress, nothing. I felt like a failure. Was I
blocking the baby? Then the contractions started again
and they were so painful that I soon took the Demerol
they offered. Afterward, the doctor walked in, donned
rubber gloves, did a vaginal exam, checked the chart and
walked out without saying a word. After several such
visits, Don followed him out of the room and insisted on

knowing what was the matter. I finally gave in and asked for the epidural. We went through the whole performance again. When the anesthesiologist returned to give me the epidural this time, it worked. They numbed me. We went to the delivery room and I kept saying, "Should I push now?" "Don't bother," was the doctor's curt answer. Meanwhile, when the doctor left the room, the nurse was guiding me and encouraging me to push and she kept telling me how well I was doing. After a short while, the doctor reappeared, saw me pushing and said, "You can push till doomsday. Nothing will happen." He never explained why. Then, without saying a word to me, he took out forceps and started to insert them. I didn't know what was happening. A resident came in and the doctor started to lecture him that the baby was turned wrong. In the mirror above me, I watched him pull on my baby's head with the forceps. It was awful. I felt so sad for my baby, and I was worried about its tiny, soft head, as the doctor tugged on it. The baby, in fact, was born with bruises on its head.

After the birth, the anesthesiologist said to Don and me, "Only one doctor in a thousand could have performed such a feat. Other doctors would have performed a caesarean." Maybe that's true, but I'm not sure. I felt the men and women attendants at the hospital were so different; the men acted like medical knowledge was a private cache. I ended up feeling helpless.

Ria and Eric were the next to report that night.

Ria and Eric

When labor started for Ria, they were wise and stayed at home as long as possible, since she was determined not to spend unnecessary hours in the hospital. Arriving at the hospital, finally, in active labor, she had to undergo routine hospital procedures: enema, intravenous drip, pubic shave. After examination by a resident, she was put to bed. At that point, her labor, too, stopped cold just as Amy's had, and they had hours of waiting without further dilation. They provided comfort for themselves by bringing some pieces of their home environment with them: a favorite quilt, some poetry, music, cards and most important, a trusted friend and Lamaze teacher to be labor coach. Somehow, the friend was able to breeze through the labor room doors with them and the three of them were ensconced there, waiting it out. Although their doctor had been told that their labor coach was coming along and was in favor of it, he hadn't cleared her presence with the hospital authorities. Consequently, he spent many of the hours during the labor battling with the power structure to allow her to remain.

> **Ria:** Fathers were accepted in the labor and delivery rooms, but a third undefined person wasn't normal, so it was a big hassle. The doctor wanted to win this political battle so that others in the future would not have the same problem.

Proud that their doctor was eager to confront the system, they nevertheless felt abandoned during his absence as he did battle, acting as guardian of the gate instead of wise counsellor-comforter during most of the labor. By the time Ria was on the delivery table, he returned and their chosen team was reunited to give her the emotional support she needed during the birth.

> **Ria:** All of us were crying for joy as the baby emerged. I was really high, even through the heavy dose of Demerol I had taken. It ended up just fine. No epidural, just Demerol. Demerol was O.K. With anything else, I wouldn't have been able to push effectively. My baby hadn't turned in the pelvis either, as Amy's hadn't, and

if I hadn't been able to push, the doctor would have had to use forceps. It would have been a far more complicated delivery. As it was, it was comparatively easy, so I'm convinced that there are things that are done in the way birth is managed that interfere with what we women do naturally.

Anne and Sam

The workshop sessions were over several months before Sam and Anne's baby was due. They had joined very early in their pregnancy. After hearing the troubling stories of their friends' hospital deliveries, they opted for a home birth. Even though their choice carried its own anxieties, they felt as though it would allow them more control over how their baby began its life.

Fortunately for them, their obstetrician, an older woman well known in her field, agreed to deliver their baby at the apartment of close friends. The friends, a couple who were both doctors, lived a few blocks from their physician's hospital. They felt very fortunate to be able to make these arrangements.

Anne's labor was prolonged. At one point, contractions recurred ten minutes apart for thirty-six hours. Then they petered out, like Amy's.

Anne: I meditated on what was going on with me, trying to sense myself. I decided it was up to me. No one could do it for me or to me. I never felt anything was wrong, just slow. Interestingly, during those three days of labor, I never experienced any of the fears I had discussed in the group, fear of death or anything else. Maybe I had worked them through.

Leni: Were you feeling comfortable with the Lamaze breathing exercises? Was the panting helpful?

Anne: Yes, that became very automatic. I didn't even stop to calculate. I thought for a while that we'd have to figure out which kind of breathing I should be doing, depending on how long the contractions were. I thought it was going to be a big head trip, but somehow, I used the breathing as I felt I needed it. It just came out. I didn't bother with focusing on a certain point or whatever; it just became a tool that was just part of me, and it worked very well.

At one point, after all those hours, the doctor thought it (the baby) was in posterior position, "Now I know why you've been putzing around for these two days," she said. "That's very common with posteriors."

I had this back pain, so I really wanted somebody there pushing on my back, and we tried the different positions Lamaze recommends for the back. That was helpful. I still wanted everyone's interaction.

Then I went into transition labor, although I wasn't really conscious of it except that my breathing started to be different. That was very painful, as it turned out. I think it was because of the posterior thing. A few times toward the end of the transition when the pain was really bad, I was having trouble staying on top of it.

After that, she examined me and said, "You're fully dilated." At that point, she and Sue were into their technical thing . . . I mean, the doctor had instruments and things, I guess an umbilical clamp and whatever. I had no desire to master what they were doing. I had such respect and trust for the two of them, that I could let them do their own thing. It is such a relief not to have to think, "Oh my God—they are down at the foot of the bed collaborating, thinking up something to do to me." It was just another example of how being at home was so fantastic. I was able to give up my whole compulsion about being part of *all* the decisions that physicians make. I felt I could really trust them, let them do their thing and take care of myself. Throughout all of this time, though, we were working together. I really very much had this sense, and I keep describing the birth as the six of us doing it.

The interaction was so smooth and so alive and it was really terrific. I just never would have gotten through this at all on my own. I never would have. I would have been too discouraged and gone to the hospital and done the Pitocin thing. But here at home, everybody was leaving it to me. Nobobdy was pushing any of their thing on me—including the physician—leaving it to me, all the way through.

Leni: It was just what you wanted. I remember you had said earlier, "I don't want people interfering with me. I want Sam there to protect me and to help make sure that what I want, I can be clear about. And if I'm not clear, I want protection so I can have time to become clear and not be messed with."

Anne: The doctor got me into incredibly active pushing. Then she withdrew and sat on the end of the bed. Sam and Sue came up and the three of us were pushing. It was so different from our practice sessions with Lamaze. In this situation, the three of us were a whole unit of energy. In between contractions, too, I was hanging onto hands—one on each side. The energy coming through the hands was really something. I just lay back and absorbed the flowing energy between contractions and then I was ready to do another.

Sam: I got to see the results of different things that we tried. I had both of my hands behind her back supporting her and I noticed after the second push that there was no progress. When I pushed with her, she pushed back very hard . . . it was all I could do to support her strength in pushing.

And I could see, I could look right down between her legs and see the baby's head push out and come back each time.

Anne: Sue would say, "I can see, it's a quarter." Then she'd say, "It's fifty cents. You've got to make it an orange." I was tuned into just everything around me and my body, too. Incredible. I just—I had partly, from video tape and a couple of films that I saw of birth, had this whole picture—I was seeing it in my head. My eyes were absolutely shut during the whole pushing thing, but I was seeing an entire scene. I knew what it looked like. Really, really marvelous. Also from inside, I was absolutely acutely aware of every sensation. For instance, between contractions, as the baby would move back deeper into the birth canal I remembered similar feelings to how he would move when he was in the womb, when he would shift his body around. I can't tell you how acute my sensations were—I was totally into that part of me, completely.

I could feel the doctor rotating his head because he had been posterior.

We decided the next pushing series would bring the baby out. I asked her whether I should be holding back after the head comes out. She said, "Yes, I'll tell you when to stop pushing." When the head came out, she said, "O.K., hold it." I was panting. I was soaking wet.

The doctor put her finger in and just turned him with a flip, pulled his head around the right way and he came out.

Sam: It was exciting. I could see the head crowning. It would appear and then disappear. What seemed to help the baby at that point, was a great deal of physical support of Anne's back. I tried to give her something strong to lean against by placing my arms and chest under her back. The force of the contractions was powerful. I had a tennis elbow for three weeks afterward, but more important than my discomfort was my feeling that I helped my baby to get born. I had a real sense of participation.

He was crying and he wasn't even out yet, and then all of a sudden he was out, and he was sitting there— this glistening light, and he *still* was crying. When he came out, he was absolutely pink.

After the birth, the doctor handed me the scissors and asked me to cut the cord. It was translucent and beautiful, with the consistency of rubber hose. I cut it slowly.

Our pediatrician friend who attended us checked our son out immediately, then Mark fell asleep in the cradle. A few hours later, he woke up and Anne was resting. I picked him up and held him in my arms as I watched the ball game. I knew he was mine. No question about that. I didn't have to see him through the window.

Ruth and Harvey

In a subsequent group, it was the first rather than the last couple to give birth who once again felt pressed into choosing a home delivery. Over several sessions, we had worked through various exercises as had the former group: a visit to the doctor and a rehearsal of the birth. The next week, Ruth and Harvey went for their appointed visit to the obstetrician armed with very specific questions. Since Harvey was a physician himself, there was added weight in his presence. They confronted the doctor with questions about routine procedures. He answered that he did require an I.V. during labor so that in case there was need for emergency medication it would be right there. Yes, he would use a fetal monitor if necessary. In fact, he told them that just the other night a baby of one of his patients would have been stillborn if he had not used the monitor. When asked about an episiotomy, he said he'd wait and see, but for the first birth it's usually a routine procedure!

> **Ruth:** I kept thinking, I sure hope he's patient. He gave very reasonable medical answers to all our questions and we kind of "yes"-ed along until we got home and started thinking it through. I began to realize that he might not even be at my birth; it might be one of his two associates. That threw me. I didn't want that at all. Sure, I had already met them. Quick introductions. In two minutes it was over. I never had the chance to talk with them. I told him I really wanted *him* to deliver the child, that I felt close to him, but he told me he couldn't promise that. However, he had arranged it so that he would be the one that I would see for my next two appointments before the due date. When it came right down to making the appointments, he was all booked up for the first and second times and I had to see the other doctors anyway. That did it! We began to plan for a home delivery. We decided we would plan to give birth at home, if the baby was in a normal position.

Since Harvey worked in a large city hospital, he felt confident that he would be able to find a physician or midwife to attend them at home. It turned out to be an almost impossible task. Their fruitless search surprised us all. Finally, they learned that the nurse who was the head of the intensive care unit at Harvey's hospital had been a midwife for many years in her native Jamaica, and she agreed to come. Ruth and Harvey were pleased at their good fortune.

Having decided to deliver at home, they invited the group members to be present, along with Ruth's parents, Harvey's son from a former marriage and several close friends.

A week later, at four P.M., Harvey called and asked me to come as soon as I could. "Ruth's in labor!"

We arrived from all over, at different intervals, most coming directly from work. My coleader, Tom, flew in from a medical meeting in Boston. Ruth's labor started in earnest at about five o'clock. The emotional energy in the room was extraordinary.

Ruth looked beautiful. She sat on the bed with her legs folded under her, rocking rhythmically through each contraction, her head and body rolling, her eyes closed, the long loose white caftan she was wearing yielding to the shape of her full breasts and moon belly.

At first, as we gathered around Ruth, there was tentativeness in each of us in such an unfamiliar circumstance. That soon passed as we became absorbed in the drama and power of the event in which we were participating. Each of us began to sense when and how to comfort Ruth by massaging or stroking her between contractions, with the midwife's sensitive guidance. Being with a couple during birth is a privileged form of sharing and each of us was conscious of that.

At eleven P.M., after six hours of intense labor, Aaron was born. At that moment, I felt we all touched eternity. It was impossible to be silent.

Awe, wonder, ecstasy, relief, joy and love mingled in a tender swelling fugue of murmuring sound. The actual words mattered not at all. The midwife placed the baby at Ruth's breast and Harvey lay down beside them on the big bed. When the cord stopped pulsating, Harvey cut it and gently immersed his new-born son in the warm bath that had been readied. Aaron was quietly alert, splashing gently, following our movements and looking attentively at each of us in the room. Soon after, Ruth delivered the placenta. Harvey wrapped the baby in a towel and, with no need for words, the room emptied, each of us sensing their need to be alone.

A week later, the words flowed freely:

Ruth: It certainly hurt a lot, especially during the last ten contractions or so, but it had its rhythm, its compelling force. There was just no way I could stop, no turning back. I just had to do it to keep moving with

it. . . . I remember saying in one of our sessions, "I
wonder what makes the baby come out? What is that
thing?" Now, I know. I read all those books about the
physical part and the medical part and the breathing
techniques and what to do with herbs and all of it.
When it came right down to it, it was *my heart* that
gave birth to the baby. It wasn't my breathing, it wasn't
the control of the breath, panting and all, it was heart
that was so strong in that room.

Having the whole group there with me was
tremendous. You know, as everyone gathered round me
for those hours, I never really knew whose hands were
stroking me; it didn't matter; it was a continuous stream
of love and reinforcement. I just remember looking up at
one point and seeing Ellen standing opposite me, her
pregnant belly quivering, her eyes filled with tears. Our
eyes met for what seemed like an eternity.

The responses from others present at the birth were colored by
the unique needs and personal expectations that each brought to
an intense experience like this one.

Ellen, the pregnant woman, and Tom, the coleader-doctor,
both expressed their reactions in some detail.

Ellen later said that being there was incredible for her:

I remember wondering about all my anxieties, about all
the questions that I thought I would be asking, like, "Is
the baby strangling or is it breathing? Is the cord around
its neck?" It all sort of went out the window when I saw
the dark spot get bigger and bigger and then it came
out. I kept thinking it's born and yet nothing official's
happening. No people running around, no equipment, no
metal, no white things. Just a warm intimate scene. All
the while, I knew that it is not going to be this particular
way for me. One part of me was thinking, on the other
hand, I'll feel safe and I'll feel that everything is going to

be all right there in the hospital. I know I can't muster
that feeling up for myself at home the way Harvey and
Ruth have, but can it be the kind of celebration it was
for them in the hospital environment? While watching
Ruth give birth, a huge burden of fear dropped off me.
It just fell away. Ruth was deeply absorbed. I knew she
was O.K. The midwife was "ironing" the perineum,
stretching it and waiting patiently for Aaron to emerge
in his own time.

It was really incredible. I felt death there as life was
beginning. It was awesome, not frightening, not morbid,
just awesome and it was O.K. To feel death was as
miraculous as to feel life. Not the death of a person, just
those absolutes, life and death, side by side, a brush with
eternity. There was a moment when he was half in
Ruth's body and half out, when his face was so blue and
the force of him was so enormous. . . . I had a feeling
that he was determining whether he was going to do it or
not, whether he was going to go the rest of the way.
There was a split second when time was
eternal . . . then it was like fast motion when it was as
if the baby decided he was going to come out.

Tom, as a doctor, had concerns that were somewhat different
from Ellen's. He reflected later:

There was so much life energy in the room—birth
energy—so much beauty—it was powerful. We must be
afraid of it in our culture, because we certainly suppress
it. Instead, our culture breeds fear into us about the
birth process and we act out of it. I was so aware of my
medical responses, that God forbid, because she was
straining and it was taking a long time—or it seemed
like a long time—something was going to go wrong and I
would have to do something about it. In fact, everything
was working just fine; Ruth was working, the baby was

working, the midwife was working. It was that natural force that my medical conditioning was prepared to turn off. I realized how we turn it off deliberately, expensively, completely. Really, it's just like that. As doctors, we are not trained to respond to good; we are trained to respond to bad and no amount of reality testing seems to convince us that bad things don't happen as often as good things. We're trained that if we do it wrong, we're going to get into trouble. If a doctor has a setback, he'll take it out on a thousand patients after that. Being at Aaron's birth was so important for me as a physician. It made me aware and appreciative of the self-regulation aspects of the life process. I realize now why people get so angry about home delivery. They are overwhelmed by the awesome quality of the life force. Of course, there are dangers. Some babies do have trouble breathing. There can be hemorrhaging, and we can be prepared for that; and even then, sometimes babies die! We must be willing to accept death as part of life. That's the ultimate risk. The risk was present in that room for each of us. It's the end as well as the beginning. It's as if the process is in reverse. I've watched people die, watched the letting go process, letting the breath out. For Aaron, it was the way it sounds in reverse, a gentle beginning sound—"Ahhh," for a few seconds, not long—then taking hold.

In addition to my personal memories of the group sessions and the births, I had hours of videotape records of our sessions. My next task, as part of my doctoral thesis project, was to create an hour-long documentary that might eventually be used as part of a prenatal counseling support system by health professionals. It was a monumental job, but I found the tapes to be very exciting and dramatic, in the sense that reviewing the material over a short time period highlighted certain patterns I hadn't noticed before. In the course of analyzing and editing the tapes, it was necessary to go over the tapes again and again. The words bounced around in my head. Over and over again, the same sentences were repeated until they were imprinted on my memory.

I was struck by the fact that each couple, early in the pregnancy, had virtually predicted the way in which labor and delivery would happen for them. They said it in many different ways at separate intervals, often unrelated to speculations about labor and delivery. In the final tape, I placed the earlier and later statements in flashback sequence—the effect was startling. This surprising observation raised the whole question of the role of self-fulfilling prophecies in affecting what happens to us. Do we decide how some events in our life will proceed and then act out these prophecies? The birth experiences of Amy and Don and Ruth and Harvey might be seen as examples of this intriguing possibility.

My insights into the nature of the individual couples' birth experiences came directly out of working closely together as a support group for so many months. I believe not only that such groups are essential, but that they are not enough. It is necessary for us to design an environment for childbearing that integrates all aspects of birth—the physiological, emotional, spiritual, medical—into people's life experiences, so that this crucial event is viewed as part of the weave of the human tapestry, a new design, and not a rent or a tear in what should be continuous and smooth.

As a result of my work with these warm, caring couples, it became clear to me that the quality of the emotional intimacy between the people involved was perhaps the most important element influencing the environment of pregnancy and birth.

Even the proponents of "natural" or "prepared" childbirth sometimes seem so intent on the virtues of their various methods that the deep emotional quality of the experience of birth is overlooked, as if that part will take care of itself. The kind of intimacy that is needed during labor and delivery doesn't spring fullblown suddenly as contractions begin. The capacity for holding each other tenderly requires slow and tender nurturing, that comes from the heart. During times of emotional stress, we discover only what has been there all the time. The crisis simply amplifies the emotions already present. It seems to me that our fears and anxieties are only fulfilled if we don't let go, can't surrender. If we can loosen the emotional knots beforehand, the necessary physiological surrender will come more easily.

Preparation for the complex emotional and physical demands of childbirth should begin long before the actual event. We have much to learn. Telling our stories—and listening—is a beginning.

VI

Patterns and Reflections: The Group Looks Back

Awareness doesn't *cause* change—awareness *is* change.

Dick

Because the workshops were designed as creative explorations rather than scientific experiments, it is neither possible nor desirable to evaluate them in scientific terms. Nor have I made any attempt to draw rigorous conclusions from the responses of the limited number of people who met with me over the years. What I offer here is a report on our work as carried out this far—one model in a developmental process, reflecting my particular intuitive psychological and environmental focus on family development during a significant normal life transition. Other groups would undoubtedly reflect their particular personalities and specific needs. In Chapter VII, I suggest some ways to start and structure groups—with or without leaders, small or large, etc.— that may be useful in helping you design the group that is best for you.

After each workshop series came to an end, I asked group members to evaluate the experience. Shortly after each birth, I personally visited as many couples as I could and we discussed their reactions to participation in the group and their feelings about the birth of their child. Their responses helped me to redesign the structure of future groups to make the process more effective.

When I decided to make this material available in a book, I knew I wanted more specific reactions and evaluations of the group process by the people who had been most involved.

Thus, six years later, I found myself trying to contact as many parents as I could locate. Some were still close enough to visit in person, others I interviewed on the phone. It was typical of our mobile American culture that parents had moved to various parts of the country: California, Pennsylvania, Maryland, Vermont, and Washington state. Some I had lost track of entirely. However, untypical of contemporary America in the '70s, among the fifteen families I contacted, only one couple was divorced. This news was extremely gratifying to me, and I hoped—although I could not assume—that their stability as families was related to the emotional support they had received during the group sessions.

During this period it became necessary for me to return to New York from my home in Northern California. Before my trip east, where most couples still lived, I sent out a questionnaire in order to stir up memories of the group experience. I was aware of how much my own life had changed in the intervening six years, and knew the parents would need a little time to recapture the emotional climate of that pregnant year. I also wanted to stimulate thinking about the broader ramifications and possible applications of what we had learned.

In the following section, I present their answers and some of my reflections on their replies. I hope this material provides useful insights, not only into the nature of the workshops, but into the pregnant year itself. These couples spent a tremendous amount of time and energy becoming aware of their changing needs before and after the birth of their children, and their present feelings about themselves and their children reflect their increased sensitivity to many issues, a sensitivity and concern that were definitely fostered by their participation in the group sessions.

Ria and Eric

After Ria finished her nursing degree, she spent weekdays in New York completing midwifery training while Eric worked full-time at his job in Massachusetts, where they lived. He has been the major caretaker of their two children (Kathy and Neil). They have since moved to the midwest, where Ria will be a midwife in a large urban hospital. Eric is the director of a national program for young mothers and fathers that teaches early parenting.

After Kathy's birth, Ria was one of the few who had responded to the original questionnaire:

> The group experience was very important to us. It gave us the opportunity to think out loud about how we wanted Kathy's birth to happen. As we listened to the others, our ideas took form, and ultimately we were able to affect our hospital experience to some degree . . . not enough, but it was something. Our doctor was affected, too. We became far better clients, were able to ask far more specific questions and were able to talk to him about our feelings, since they were brought to a conscious level. We also affected the hospital. I nursed Kathy on the delivery table . . . a first in that hospital. They won't forget us in a hurry. I hope that softened the way for others.
>
> We both find the question, "What did you get out of the group?" so difficult to answer . . . what happened to us was such a complex experience, which we've not fully analyzed. Summarizing seems almost impossible.
>
> I had become interested in the psychology of pregnancy through my schoolwork, and also felt there were issues to be dealt with by the pregnant couple, which could be handled well in a group. I still had a rather vague sense that Eric and I were not enjoying our pregnancy as much as we might.
>
> For years I had been told by a gynecologist that I would probably not be able to conceive without intervention or medication or surgery, so I was immensely pleased to find myself pregnant. But, as the pregnancy was not planned, and began just as Eric's mother was dying, and since he was reluctant to have a

baby until I finished nursing school, I was worried about how things would work out for us as a couple.

I didn't know what I felt should be happening, but so much of the time I felt the pregnancy was just within me . . . rather than within us . . . and that was a lonely feeling, a frightening one. I didn't know what was wrong, but felt that something definitely was not right, and so looked to the group that our friend talked about, as a chance for Eric and me to be more fully together.

As I look back, I realize how little I knew of what was missing. It was only through the group, which released us to fulfill so much more of our potential for sharing, that Eric and I learned how far apart we had been.

What happened to me in the group was, I think, a general sort of release. Eric and I began to talk more and more, and to work together in planning for the birth and child care. The feelings I'd had inside me all along (positive and negative) found their ways into words, and in sharing with others, I discovered new ideas and feelings about pregnancy and birth, and children and parenting. It was terribly exciting, and a strengthening experience for me. My loneliness subsided a good deal . . . I-we became more alive and open to pregnancy, with its joys and deepest fears.

And yet we didn't really deal with the issue of Eric's anger about the unplanned pregnancy, nor with the question of whether I was to blame for that event. We must have talked all around it without ever looking at this issue straight on. And it has continued to be a source of tension and mistrust in our relationship, which we are just now beginning to try to explore.

I had no idea that Eric was as angry as he was about the unplanned baby, nor that he felt I'd tricked him into pregnancy. I wished that I had been able to open up about it in the group instead of holding back, when I had the opportunity.

* * *

Six years after Kathy's birth, Ria responded in her usual thoughtful detail to my second questionnaire:

We *have* recommended group experiences to people going through various pregnancies—that is, we've often talked about our group and the value it had for us, and encouraged people to put together their own support groups, especially if childbirth education classes aren't meeting their needs. The fact is that such groups are not usually available, and they need to be started. My current idea is that once I get settled in a job as a staff midwife, Eric and I can teach childbirth classes together and create a group experience along the lines of the group we had with you. A group that deals with the whole experience of being pregnant and giving birth, becoming a family. I know that we needed your group (our group) quite apart from our preparation for childbirth series, and there was more work to do than could be fit in around the relaxation exercises, etc.—but as a midwife, I really don't see how one can do the one without the other. . . .

I think a similar group would have been great for our pregnancy with our second child. The openness was there again, some of the same issues were asking to be dealt with, and there were certainly as many changes to be coped with as the first time around—different ones, but as many. It's really a matter of taking advantage of a unique time for growth as individuals and as a couple— as a family, too. . . . We were so concerned about Kathy's sharing in Neil's birth, and as I will probably tell you somewhere down the line, it was surprising to find how little we had prepared *ourselves* for the change in her life.

Yes, indeed, if we were pregnant again, we would both want a group.

Yes, I would recommend a book on the group to friends. Perhaps it might be difficult for a lot of people to do the exercises on their own, but they might be moved more strongly to put together a group, find a facilitator, if they had a book as a guide.

The most difficult aspect of my first pregnancy was dealing with the relationship between Eric and me. We became pregnant with a lot going against us, I think: unplanned pregnancy; me in school and Eric's mother terminally ill with leukemia (she died when I was two months pregnant).

The list could probably go on, but this is enough! At any rate, much of this was just simmering away in each of us, not being talked about very much, not being dealt with in any productive way, and giving rise to a lot of anger which came out in other ways, creating a lot more tension between us.

I remember worrying because Eric never brought up the subject of the pregnancy, never wanted to touch my belly. I was basically pleased to be pregnant (though not without a lot of mixed feelings). I remember Lucy Ann's suggesting the group, and then suggesting it myself to Eric. My memory is that he was reluctant at first but agreed to do it. That was when we began to be pregnant *together*. We had the one night a week which we saved for ourselves, for the pregnancy and the baby and trying to come to grips with what was happening to us.

It was so incredibly important that we had the baby together. I look back on the experience and can see all kinds of problems which had to be worked out later on, but we made progress then, and I think if we hadn't we might well not have gotten through the even harder (in some ways) times ahead for us as a couple.

The easiest and most joyful aspect of the pregnancy was the physical experience of carrying a child, and then the actual childbirth. And then, I think, *the* most joyful aspect of the entire process was falling in love with

Kathy, and with ourselves as a family—but that has been for us a gradual process, a growth into more excitement and joy. It certainly didn't happen immediately when she was born, although we were both very thoroughly engrossed in her from the beginning. I found the hospitalization lonely, uncomfortable emotionally and sometimes physically, too, full of annoying routines—but I also have a very special feeling about that time: the smell of Vaseline, the Jamaican voices, my baby being wheeled in during the night to be nursed and then just curled up on my bare chest afterwards to sleep; my body going through all those enormous changes, all normal and purposeful and deeply exciting to me.

Eric: We came into the group after being "recruited" by a friend. We didn't know much about what the group would involve, but expected an expansion of the Lamaze material. In retrospect, for me Lamaze appears to need a great deal of expansion, and the group showed clearly how many issues are not explored in the skill-oriented Lamaze sessions. Lamaze feeds right into the technology of the hospital—an approach not broad enough to encourage more creative dealing with the complex questions involved in childbearing.

Earlier, I felt tricked into having a baby. . . . Ria had wanted it, not me. . . . When the group began, I was having a hard time thinking about the baby at all or about myself as a father. I'd considered our pregnancy helpful not for me but for my father, giving him a "life" focus after my mother's recent death. But that wasn't me. One of the major impacts of the group on me was that it forced me to think of myself as a father and permitted me to think about my fathering fantasies. . . . In the course of the workshop, I moved from not having thought much about the baby at all to saying that I wanted a major part of the responsibility for childcare after the birth. Actually, the group experience facilitated expression of my ideas about involvement. They were part of me, I know, but might never have been expressible or capable of development unless I had them shared with others.

Elena and Dick

Elena is a social worker with a poetic bent. After the birth of their first daughter, Becky, she started to do some personal writing, some of which has since been published. Dick is an architect who works for a large design firm. They are still living in New York.

Elena and Dick's new baby daughter, Ellie, was three months old when I visited them in New York some years later.

Elena: I think I'm quite different with this baby, and that makes her different. I guess I trusted my feelings more this time. I also feel we're more mature.

Dick: It's true. We didn't talk about it a lot this time, but I was more aware of your feelings. However, I didn't talk about my feelings this time. Actually, you did. Do we use each other in this way? Yes, I think that old pattern still holds. If you worry, then I don't have to and vice versa. . . . We divide up the issues of concern and collude together—when you worry, I have to be the caretaker.

Elena: We were very involved without our own parents during the first time . . . psychologically. I really wanted my mother around that first pregnancy, I remember. She came but stayed with her sister. Maybe I should have been more explicit about asking her to stay with me. Then she fell down on the way over to see me and arrived bleeding, needing my help just when I needed her! Her solution was to call up her twin sister and ask her to come instead. Even though she didn't do these nice motherly things like get tea, I wanted *her*. Then it was amazing. . . . She said, "I know how scared you are," and that opened up a lot. Since she was not giving me what I needed, I had to get it somewhere else.

But I have trouble asking people for help. In my childhood, I recall my mother saying, "Neither a borrower nor a lender be." I realized during this pregnancy that I was basically alone. At the same time, I also knew that I could get what I needed if I was grown up about handling it. I realized that was what maturity was about. Maturity is learning that you can make your own choices.

I never thought of it as a therapy group, though I suppose it was. I think when you call it a support group, it's much less threatening. You're very vulnerable when you're pregnant and getting "therapized" is a scary thought, though one may need exactly that. If you call it a support group, then you can explore just what a support group is.

You know, you need a lot of mothering during pregnancy. The father needs it, too. Dick let his feelings out more than most men but he got neglected by me. In the group, men got paid attention to. Did you ever consider that we think it's terrific if a pregnant woman's mother comes to take care of her daughter and makes it easier, especially during and after the birth, but no man's mother rushes over to take care of her son! He needs a lot, too. In fact, the final straw may be that the mother-in-law rushes over to take care of her daughter-in-law.

Dick: It's true this time I felt even more excluded. Last time, I wanted to run away. Maybe this time there was a letdown because the group was not there. Elena was self-contained. It took me a while to realize that might be a problem for me. And the last thing I wanted was to disturb her sense of security.

Elena: And I felt grabby about the experience. I wanted it for myself.

Dick: Maybe I envy you more than I ever acknowledge. What an experience! I tend to run issues out in the abstract. I take pleasure in someone else's accomplishments rather than envy them.

It strikes me that the group was such a special setting for me because it was one of the few places where we knew that someone would listen to the next thing we would say, no matter what it was. We knew it wouldn't be just tolerated, but the attempt to understand would be made in an open-minded way. My confidence in that allowed me to go on to say the next thing. . . . I might not have been able to do that otherwise.

Elena: In other groups, others are always waiting to say their thing.

Dick: It's true. I know in most group situations, I like to be the center of attention. I suppose everyone does. It was much easier to deal with her because I knew that the quality of attention given to each person would eventually be focused on me, too.

I was never bored. People were sharing quite honestly, sharing deep parts of themselves. I found their concerns related to me. I was always learning something from what was happening and so I didn't feel impatient about listening to others.

I had an awful lot of ambivalence about our coleader, Tom. In particular, about being manipulated—of being plugged into a system that was not of my own making. I'm used to working with systems, but I had a terror getting in touch with my own feelings. Now, I'm more comfortable if someone says, "This process will get you in touch with your emotions."

Leni: Why were you more suspicious of Tom than of me?

Dick: Because Tom was a man. I had to take him seriously. I was used to being manipulated by my mother. I knew how to handle that—or at least I had a system for that. And my father had bullied me.

Leni: Did being in the group help you with the second pregnancy?

Dick: I didn't have a romantic sense about birth this time around. It was a more peaceful, steadier feeling. The earlier group experience was very helpful in helping that happen. It relaxed me. Would I have put earphones on Elena's abdomen unless we had done those exercises dialoguing with the baby? At the time I felt very foolish, writing that letter to the person in the womb. But it was an icebreaker—a party game. Even as I did it, there was a spine-tingling sense that there was a person inside and that I could contact it.

Elena: The exercises did threaten me. I was in therapy. I felt safe there and I didn't want you to threaten that relationship. I was pretty angry with you, Leni, a lot of the time. I felt you shouldn't have been involved in this kind of group leadership because you weren't a professional or credentialed. Tom was, *he* was a doctor. I felt pressured to have this ideal birth. You said I had control. I didn't see that I did. But I valued the male/female co-leadership a lot . . . it was really important. I had always gone to women to share my feelings. And my therapist was a woman. I liked the fact that Tom was a doctor, even though he wasn't an ob-gyn. It made me feel comfortable and confident. He also shared a lot of himself. And being in the group with fathers and role playing a visit to the doctor with their participation helped me deal with the second birth and the doctor I had this time. Incidentally, he could have done me in but I didn't let him. This time, I had a vaginal birth, even though the first one was a caesarean.

Dick: Tom was a wonderful model for me because he was soft inside. I hadn't given it much conscious thought before the group experiences. My ambition was to feel and to express the feminine part of me. I realized that philosophically I believed that, but in practice I suppressed it. Male role models in my life haven't emphasized that.

Elena: I do think most people have their babies for specific intellectual reasons which may mask the unconscious ones. I never thought about it, but I am a "Show me" person. It's hard for me to take risks. Having a baby and writing a book were great risks. I was struggling with my identity at the time. I didn't feel I had any professional identity; everything was unresolved for me at the time of the group. I kept thinking, how can Leni say she is a professional when *I* can't? She's just working on her doctorate.

Do you remember my dream about the garbage? I was letting go of the need for credentials . . . finding out who I was.

Dick: It's interesting, Elena, that the book you went on to write paid honor to exactly that "anticredentialed" mode. And that even your therapist was not credentialed.

Elena: It's true—I've changed more in the past five years than in my whole life—no, in the past three years. . . .

Dick: I learn by taking the risk of asking, and through the experience of what happens next.

I think a lot of what's been happening to me began
with the group and through the exercises, but it was
with the arrival of the child that I began to articulate
what was going on, and bring together my intellect and
my feelings.

I've never been happier than I am now. It's a
challenge and it gives me a lot of energy. That's what
therapy is about . . . freeing energy.

I've gone into therapy since then. I was getting
increasingly unhappy in my work. I wasn't allowed to do
things I needed to do. I am well on the way now to
becoming my own person. I began to suppress my
intuitive abilities. Now I know I have to meld and
balance these two aspects of myself.

Change is our human goal, our collective striving.
What does our role contribute to generate change, to
expand, to take on the universe? Customarily, we have
thought in terms of physical expansion but it is psychic
and psychological as well.

Dick is changing. He is becoming father to himself as
well as to his children instead of simply son to his
father.

Leni: What could be done to make the groups even
more effective?

Elena: The tribe doesn't prepare you for parenting. It
used to be a secret about motherhood. At least now you
can talk about it. A pregnancy group needs to
incorporate the postbirth period, too. It's an out of joint
time. I tried to escape from it. It would have been nice
to anticipate the stresses there as well.

I would like to have a group that followed through
the birth and early parenting. In the group we had
established a support system and we needed each other
afterwards. We needed the people we had shared our

deep feelings with, people we could continue to be
honest with. We had a hard time at the beginning. Once
you have one baby, you forget the early stuff that
seemed so important. But the issues remain to be
resolved differently with each child.

Jean and Paul

Jean and Paul were in one of the groups. They were divorced
two years ago, after twelve years of marriage. Jean has continued
her career as an interior designer and has become quite successful.
Paul is a management consultant. They continue to live within
blocks of each other in New York City so that their son, Josh, can
see his father on weekends, and frequently during the week. I
visited Jean during the summer after seeing Ria and Eric.

Jean: I don't know where I was career-wise then, but
it's really flourishing now. I'm doing things I really want
to do. When Josh was eighteen months old, I got very
involved in designing residences and offices and since
then I have been very busy.
   Paul and I split up when Josh was just over three.
Being a single parent is hard and it's been important for
Paul and me to maintain a good relationship. We've
known each other a long time. We were very young when
we met and married.
   The value of the group is hard to verbalize; it's much
more in the gut than anywhere. There are so many
things that only make sense later.
   Being in a group with other people who were sharing
the same experience put me in touch with the fact that I
was part of a universal process. My words then, come
back to me now. I had never considered before that my

mother had given birth and her mother before her had given birth to her, that it was an endless stream. I suppose it felt like stepping over a barrier to be reunited with humanity—a totality was realized. That's where the group came into it.

Being with others who were going through the same thing, talking about our history . . . our parents' experience, even our grandparents' experience and about pregnancy and birth as an initiation rite provoked the image of stepping over a barrier. The barrier? Let's see, if it was in a dream, there would be a conveyor belt and several people along the side standing still, then one hopping in every so often. . . . The belt would be endless.

Leni: Is that the life stream?

Jean: Yes. During the pregnancy, I guess I indulged myself so much that I really, really dreamed. I loved my body so much. I loved my pregnancy so much. I think I would want another child, just to be pregnant again. I can't remember feeling bad. I remember feeling how my body felt inside. I think I was more in touch with my center, my physical center, than ever before. And that barrier I talked about had a lot to do with reality, too.

I think I would probably say that the people who were standing there, getting in touch with the flow were women—it was just women on the conveyor belt who were being initiated into the rights of womenhood.

Leni: Could the group be more in touch with that process? Should the groups be just women?

Jean: No, I kept hoping the other men would show Paul how I wanted him to feel. In retrospect (because I wouldn't allow myself to recognize it at the time), I think I became more aware of the differences between my husband and me. I remember feeling upset with some of his views and at the same time feeling guilty at being critical because it should have been a time of togetherness.

Leni: You never got mad.

Jean: Perhaps I might have worked through more of those feelings in the group but I really don't think there was anything to be done about the marriage.

The group experience was helpful. You get some clarity and validation for how you're feeling when you see how others are behaving and responding to you. It was also easier for Paul to see things as they were when he observed it objectively. I guess it was George who really identified with being jealous about what went on in a woman's body. I loved the fact that a man could express those feelings because I'm sure that a lot of men feel that same thing. I liked that Paul could be exposed to how other men felt. It's a major pitfall in a marriage though, because you want your partner to be the way you want them to be instead of seeing them the way they are.

I don't know about the exercises for me. I hadn't had any previous group experience so it felt like a foreign language—a little gimmicky. I would have preferred more talking. I got as much out of the conversation as I did out of the exercises—that is, looking at my expectations in relation to what others had experienced. It is true that a lot of feelings got stirred up, but there didn't seem to be an outlet for the feelings. Maybe it was just me not being able to deal with my feelings.

Leni: We probably needed to have private sessions with each couple at intervals also, but that would have involved a longer time commitment than you had made.

Jean: Maybe it would be better for everyone to be in private therapy concomitantly, or maybe it would just have been better for me. Now that I am in therapy and have been for three years, I can get in touch with the

feelings I had then. . . . I can know how angry I was
then at certain times and how painful it was.

Paul and I had very strong feelings for each other,
but our marriage didn't work.

I know I would have been absolutely crushed if Paul
hadn't been there at the birth. I think if it hadn't been
for the group, we would have had a harder time.

What impressed me the most was the way in which
each couple predicted the way their birth would be.
What that says to me is that each of us has the power to
control the experience to some degree. That's the one
thing that stands out for me.

It would be nice to recapture the excitement of a
second birth by being in another group. People seem so
much less intense about a second birth. The group
makes it so much more than just having a child, you are
brought into the mainstream of society. I know I would
be much more carefree about a second child. Right after
Josh was born, I remember washing my hands every
time I picked him up!

Amy and Don

Amy has pursued her career as a weaver and works full-time at
her studio in downtown Manhattan. Don teaches economics. They
take equal responsibility for childcare of their son. They have
maintained a friendship with one of the couples from their
group.

Don: Even though it wasn't planned, we were delighted.
I was very glad it was going to happen. There wasn't any
hesitation, no turning back.

Amy: You were less hesitant . . . you were forty . . . .

Don: Pregnancy is such an "up" time, unless of course, one or the other is against it, though obviously, there are some apprehensions, too. If there are personality issues that get in the way like expectations, desires, it's O.K. for them to get put aside, because giving birth—carrying on the next generation—may be the most important task we ever do and the most important experience of our lives.

The idea that you need support for the pregnancy stage feels like carrying coals to Newcastle.

Leni: It's nice to see that you're now so secure about your fathering abilities, Don, because you sure felt a lot more vulnerable back then. How well do you remember the group? For instance, what about the exercises? Were they useful?

Don: If I think back, I don't remember the exercises. I remember the people very vividly, what they said and how they related to each other, I only remember what we were *talking* about. In particular, what others were talking about, not even what I was talking about. . . . I don't know whether that is selective memory.

Amy: I do recall the exercises—I think they helped us express some problems that were difficult. I remember we had a fight about competing over this child that hadn't even been born yet. There is still some of that between us. However, I think we focus on him rather than competing with each other.

Don: I think that happened long after the birth.

Amy: No, it was there in anticipation.

Leni: Do you remember that when you talked in the group, Don would listen thoughtfully and give you a lot of support? He would sit next to you, quite obviously admiring you, playing with your hair, twirling a stray lock, giving you the very attention that you felt that you weren't receiving?

Amy: I know, that has continued. I realize he spends a lot of time looking at me and I'm not aware of it.

I've been weaving since the birth and I've had my own studio for two years. Leaving school and starting to work by myself was a trauma for me. It was almost impossible to do anything at first. It was physically difficult for me to get my whole self into it and I still don't have my whole self into it, but I'm more into it than I was two years ago. There's just this tremendous fear. It feels like this is the big test. . . . .

Leni: You are saying the same thing about fear and the big test, as you did during the pregnancy in relation to the birth.

Amy: Am I? So much of it has to do with lack of information, that's why it was so huge. Every step of the way is in the dark . . . birth, nursing, childcare.

Leni: Often so much of that information is inside you. It's allowing yourself to know what you already have sensed intuitively.

Amy: I'm starting to have a glimmer of that now, in my work.

Don: The most valuable part of the group was making the whole thing less mysterious, since we had no idea what to expect—particularly in relation to the medical community. Our experience was despicable. The whole idea of deferring to the doctor was the big shock of the whole experience. Because we went through the experience with the group, we knew that our experience was despicable. In the group, you came to trust your own judgment more about what pregnancy should be.

Our problem was with the medical profession. . . .

Even today, I still have that problem—I went to a doctor to have him look at a mole . . . he said it was a wart. When I asked him what the difference was, he said, "I don't have time to explain." The same old stuff, just like Amy's doctor saying she can push till Doomsday and it won't make any difference and not bothering to explain. How dare he say that? Nothing's changed.

As we talked in the group, you had less input, Leni, than any of the people there. I was interested in the psychology of Alan and Dick and Eric and others, but you and Lucy Ann [a nurse] had a lot of information that we never got. You were eliciting information from us, eliciting our feelings but you were the expert and should have been telling us.

Amy: My general memory is one of resentment that we were giving you a lot. I guess it was my fear of being controlled or of losing control over this experience, because it was such a nice pregnancy and because I was so ignorant of the process . . . and of what happens. Even the childbirth classes seemed to explain nothing, give no variables, no experiences of anyone else. It was really like jumping off a cliff. I knew nothing. But you knew a lot and so did Lucy Ann. You knew doctors, you knew other situations, but you never told me any of that. And you could have. You could have told me, he shouldn't be treating you like this, instead of saying, "How do you feel about him treating you this way? There are doctors who don't treat you like this." But that wasn't your purpose, you were there to transcribe, to take notes.

Amy: I didn't find out anything there, though. No one told us about our bodies. . . . They just said read this book. . . . Go there.

Leni: Do you remember seeing the videotape in which

you two were reporting about your office visits and complaining about your doctor?

Amy: I do remember talking about the doctor all the time.

Leni: We spent a lot of time on the issue of your feelings about your doctor. You didn't seem to want to hear me or others say anything about changing doctors. "Why are you going to that doctor?" . . . Eric said impatiently one night, "There are better doctors, you are getting fucked over by that doctor." It was said several times at different intervals by many members of the group. And now, years later, as we talk I'm hearing a repetition of attitude and, in fact, the same kind of language you used before.

Amy: What attitude?

Leni: The doctor is the expert; that he knows best. Don said then, "I respect doctors; they know what they are doing." I'm a professional and I respect professional training. All of us "professionals," including Lucy Ann, who was a nurse, and Ria, who was in nursing school, would say, "Look, doctors don't know everything. You may have to shop around until you find one that really suits you. But you seemed to want to stay with the one you had and be mad, instead of switching to someone more satisfying. I recall that very specifically because I was feeling frustrated. I didn't know how far to go with advice, how much to comfort you. I was consciously *not* replacing the doctor as an authority—you were angry at me for not playing into that dynamic, for not taking control. I didn't want to make decisions for you. That was not my role. I was trying to help you to hear yourself and trust your own feelings.

Don: The doctor was a forceps man, and we didn't even know what a forceps was.

Amy: I couldn't even conceive of changing doctors. It's one thing to feel that the doctor is fucking you over, another for you to tell me that I should go see this new doctor or recommend someone.

It was wonderful to have that companionship in the group; that was great. There were ties formed there. I would have liked us to be even closer to each other, to have been more of a community. I'm glad that I did it. I would have liked to have done more things like the dialogue with the baby. I remember that so vividly. Pregnant women are always communicating with their child, but this was deeper. I really transcended my own neurotic worries, and drew out some realness in me that doesn't come out very often. I think becoming a mother has changed me for the better.

I also wish there had been more touching of other pregnant women. It would have been good for men to have had more touching, too.

Anne and Sam

Anne and Sam moved to California after the birth of their first child, Mark. Anne was a management consultant. She's now doing graduate work in medical anthropology, with emphasis on children. Sam is an airlines executive, as he was during the group. They moved because Sam's firm sent him to the west. Their second son, Ted, was born nine months ago. Both children were born at home, one in New York and one in California.

Both Anne and Sam felt that the most positive aspect of the group was its effect on the development of their own relationship.

Anne: As I sat and listened to us in the group, I realized

195

that Sam and I had led separate lives for the past seven years. Our work took us into different worlds and as we pursued our careers and traveled about we were involved with different people in quite different fields. I hadn't understood how separate we were.

Sam: This was the first important thing we faced together.

Anne: We had to come to grips with working things out in common, doing some problem-solving together. The process of drawing together was very powerful for me and is still quite clear to me six years later. I recall we sat there drawing on one piece of paper. I felt in touch with nature and organic function; I drew a large tree. There was no person in my image, however. When Sam came along and put in the person, I scratched out the figure Sam was drawing. I was annoyed. I didn't want a person messing up my image of nature. Imagine! I realize when I remember those feelings that having people in the group who were further along than I was, helped make my pregnancy seem more real earlier on. I needed to accept it, not continue to feel that it was a movie, and not happening to me.

Sam: I remember that Anne was quite ambivalent in the early months, not about having the baby, which she wanted—but about accepting all the complexities of the social changes that subsequently occur. It took time to work that through to a comfortable place. The group helped us focus on important things that had to develop in our relationship as a couple so that we would be in a good place to welcome the new person. We began to realize what it is like to have a baby.

We listened a lot to how others felt. There was a rare depth of sharing with the others. We understood more about how we ourselves had been treated and how that patterned our lives. We felt much better prepared as a result. Our relationship is closer than it has ever been.

Anne: In the second birth, I felt Sam's total support. The experience in the group probably helped him do that. And now with our second baby, we sit down and talk about our differences in attitudes about childbearing. . . . We have come together around the children.

Sam: I can't truly recall specific exercises, or even the exercises in general or the feelings I had during them. I did like the structure of the evenings and enjoyed the group. It was very important to us.

Anne: I liked the exercises. In fact, recently I wanted some help to look once again at issues that arose. Some were the same and I wanted to go into them more deeply. I went to various groups for help, tried to start a parent group with fathers as well as mothers. No luck! Finally, I organized a support group which met every third week. When I was trying to plan some sessions for this group of parents, I used some of the exercises from our group and from other exercises I'd had. It's an art to apply them to the right moment. I feel you did that well in our group. I felt they were facilitative.

There is no place to get in touch with the feelings during pregnancy. In childbirth classes, they say education will take care of the fear but they don't deal with it. Letting myself feel vulnerable was my personal task. It was the first time I could let myself do it. I prided myself on my great strength before out in the man's world. I feel that to be a key issue in the contemporary world—allowing the feelings of vulnerability to be there instead of being in control and invulnerable. Surrendering. That's what one learns in therapy or I did, anyway . . . allowing oneself to be sad, to be in pain, to feel fear . . . it's all part of life. I recall one in which we focused on a light that circulated around the baby and after we relaxed we were asked to talk to the baby.

It was important to me to deal with the baby as a person, important to deal with its consciousness from the start. It was simple but profound. I have recommended that exercise to many pregnant friends. It's odd to recall all this now. I was surprised at how much more acceptance Sam had for having a child. He connects with the kids on a deep level; he's a good father. He doesn't have a lot of close adult friends, so it's a side I hadn't seen.

I do remember that I didn't feel as close to the group as I wanted to. I think I would have liked more socializing in between. And yet the support they gave us was essential.

We never would have done a home birth without the group. I discovered that I had choices, that it was important for me to arrange things the way I wanted them to be. The group gave us the impetus to design our birth environment as we dealt with all the issues of designing one's birth in the group. Hearing the horrors of others' experiences convinced me that we had to have it at home.

Sam: Now that I look back at our first home birth, I realize that we were so lucky. Things fell into our laps . . . the compliance of our traditional OB, the support of our two best friends, who were both doctors and offered us their home for the birth which was close to the hospital. In California, the region of home births, strangely, it was hard to find help for the second birth. If we had had to push as hard to organize the first as we did the second, we wouldn't have done it. It was so great the first time that we did persevere.

Anne: I find the women's movement is still putting down motherhood right and left. The most difficult aspect of my life has been integrating my commitment outside in the world and inside the domestic realm. The group could help me find my true feelings, which were

that I needed to go with family as long as that was
necessary although I didn't get specific help on that
issue. But, in actuality, I had to hear from a man I really
trusted that it was all right to have a family as first
priority. My male colleagues were saying to me, "My
wife is so miserable. Don't choose to stay home." I'm
happy I chose to have a family, and Sam and I are
struggling with how we each participate in the domestic
realm. The world needs to help men get the joy that is
inherent in creating and shaping lives. We're working at
the parenting process. We had no idea of what parenting
would be like. I now have a whole notion that you
develop as the child develops. Things are different in
contemporary America.

The transpersonal aspects of birth were closer to me
this time, permitting me to feel the spiritual presence. It
has been most powerful for me and Sam. We chose a
quotation from Lao-Tzu to say it for us for the
welcoming of our second child. We wanted something
besides baptism which is a ceremony that washes away
the sin from the sinful arrival of the baby. I was feeling
just the opposite . . . how do we keep the purity of this
being?

The breath of life moves through a deathless valley
Of mysterious motherhood
Which conceives and bears the universal seed,
The seeming of a world never to end,
Breath for men to draw from as they will:
And the, more they take of it, the more remains.
Lao-Tzuo
The Way of Life
(translated by Witter Bynner)

We needed you the second time, Leni. I wish we had

been able to be with you in a group for that time. You
know I called you to see if you could put it together even
for a weekend. Let me send you a journal entry from my
second pregnancy—the learning goes on, you know.

August 7, starting last trimester:
"I want to write about what went on for me about a
month ago, after I got back from New York. When I
visited good friends there, I was feeling very positive
about my life now—the prospect of graduate work,
which I've already embarked on and am feeling
productive about; the coming baby, which delights Sam
too; Sam and I are at a good level of caring and
acceptance; Mark is lovely; our new home is wonderfully
restorative, a joy to be in; we are basically healthy;
Sam's job is going very well. So I exuded this aura of
competence, and genuinely felt it.

"Then I came home, was glad to be home, but
realized I was walking around with all this anger—at
everyone, even the shopkeepers, other drivers, the whole
world, in fact. Just all-pervasive anger.

"I let my irrational self express it, and here's what it
said, loud and clear: 'I want to be taken care of.' It was
an overwhelming feeling, all pervasive, totally vulnerable
and needy. I want a mother and father. I want someone
to take care of me at the birth, and before and after.

"Well, I still get in touch with this level of feeling
from time to time. Probably I'll never lose it and maybe
it's a human dimension. Who says I have to be
competent all of the time? I still want to be held
sometimes. Mainly, I have to let myself feel vulnerable;
just acknowledging the feeling really helps a lot, and it
helps connections with other people who are also in
need.

"I'm less demanding. I'm closer to Mark and Sam.
But it is painful, too.

"I suspect pregnancy intensifies these feelings of vulnerability, though they are always present in us, just usually buried really deep, under the anger and control."

Rachel and Alan

Rachel conceived during the last month of the group and gave birth at a birth center, one of the few in the Pacific Northwest, the region of her own birth. Rachel and Alan have stayed in the Northwest, where Alan has been the doctor for a small community for the past four years. During the period of the group workshop, he was completing his residency in a large New York hospital.

Rachel is busy as a homemaker and helping to develop the farmland they have bought and taking care of their daughter, Susie. When I saw them they were expecting their second child, who was due in six months.

It was eight months after the group had ended when their first baby was born. They called me to share their excitement. They had driven to their birth center at ten A.M. with the majestic sight of the mountains before them. As the sun was setting at five-fifty-five P.M., Susie was born. The birth center was a perfect place for Rachel to give birth.

Rachel: The environment was like a home and full of mementos. Contractions went fast, the midwife was a sweet, beautiful woman, a perfect person to have there. I felt so happy to see her. Alan was there and felt a little jealous and left out because this woman was so special to me. Later we talked about it and it was O.K. The second stage took longer and was a little complicated but it worked out. I felt irritated at some points that the baby was so difficult and disappointed to have to have an episiotomy.

During labor I felt so earthbound, nothing else
mattered. It was an all-encompassing experience.
Nothing else mattered. Alan didn't matter, just giving
birth. I thought at one point, "I'm not getting spiritual
enough," but in retrospect, there was a glow about it. I
didn't need bells or music. It was extraordinary.

Alan: Early on during labor, I felt she needed a servant,
not me, just someone to fetch and carry. I felt resentful.
I wanted it to be a peak experience to her. I heard it was
such a high, but how do you absorb this life experience
in such a little time? But it was magical.

It's difficult to bring ourselves mentally back to that
time, to be able to easily discuss the birth group. That
emotional state is worlds away. Our lives have changed
so much, I am no longer who I was then—my marriage
and practice aren't the same and yet it's timely that you
have asked us just now, because Rachel's pregnant with
our second child—you're one of the few people who
know now. We feel that we would like to keep this one a
secret for a few months—something to be experienced
just by us at first before we spring it on the
grandparents and friends.

Rachel: The first time I was pregnant we were going to
be homeless for quite a while and it was quite different.
Now we're part of a community and we're going to be
around for the next many months.

Alan: Pregnant women get a little of what I get as a
doctor. I can't even go to social occasions on the island
without being assailed by questions and personal
problems—I've started to avoid parties, even though I
used to be very gregarious.

Rachel: We had to become secure enough in our
relationship to feel O.K. enough about bringing someone
else into our family. A lot of my concern was due to the
fact that my parents were divorced and that caused me a

lot of distrust in relationships. I was finally able to feel confident enough in our relationship to go ahead.

Alan: We both take the idea of marriage very seriously—which made us very frightened of the responsibility that we were taking—in terms of the commitment that we made. Also frightened that if we didn't do it right, it wouldn't work, because all around us people were having trouble with their relationships. At times it seemed like everybody was. There we were even before we had a baby wondering whether it was the right thing to do and it seemed like Rachel didn't get pregnant until it was right for it to happen. Even now, sometimes we wonder. . . .

Rachel: You have to have a firm base because there are all kinds of tests. There's that complication of another person. It does make marriage a lot more difficult. We have moved a lot in time and space, though, by coming to this community. I can't imagine a farther place to be from where we were in Manhattan—in both environment and culture, at least in the United States. It's so different being in a city of several million to being in a town of several thousand. . . . We're still surrounded by water, though.

Alan: We've changed so many of our ideas. Some of our old ideas seem to us so naïve now. That's the way it goes. I was such a radical—a revolutionary—but in becoming a father I realized I didn't want to bring a child up in chaos. It seems consistent to see young people who are just getting married who are so idealistic.

Rachel: I think I already feel a qualitative difference with this pregnancy. I don't mean that the magic is not there, I'm sure I'll feel the same as I did, but we were on a cloud the first time. We had bought a dulcimer just to play music for the baby while we drove across the country. That's great, but I'm much more practical now.

You asked about how the exercises helped and what impact they had. I remember one in particular. We were acting out going to the doctor's office and stating what we wanted. That helped me a lot because when we came out here I hadn't had any continuous medical care. I had just stopped on the way and had various people examine me. I was about five months pregnant and very healthy. I had a lot of expectations for the birth. Fortunately, I found a birth center out here. I went into the birth center armed with all these questions—and very determined. Working together with the group in New York helped me formulate and verbalize my ideas. Having practice helped. It turned out not to be necessary because the midwife in the clinic was anxious to do what parents wanted.

Alan: When it came to deciding where we would have the baby, I was less anxious to have it in a birth center than in a hospital—the hospitals in this area are not like big city hospitals with their cold, steely environments. Of course, hospitals here are not the same quiet, personal places that perhaps a birth center or home is but they are much more geared towards families and natural childbirth. They have rooms that are set aside for this kind of birth—different from those we had left, where midwives had to be hired furtively in order for women to have babies that way. I'm sure things have changed in other parts of the country by now. This birth center has helped to pioneer new ways. We were fortunate, but even so, I wasn't that eager because I was concerned about the risks.

Rachel: I want to have the baby at the same birth center. But I'm also not that opposed to the hospital. I'd be willing to go look, whereas before I would only have been willing to go if I couldn't have the birth center—I don't feel so threatened by the hospital now, maybe because I know some of the doctors now and I trust them.

Leni: Do you feel different about this pregnancy?

Alan: It's again a transition time—but we'll be living here for some time. We're remodeling our house now and will probably just be taking off the roof and beginning phase two when the baby is born.

Rachel: There's no perfect time to have a baby.

Alan: Getting back to the value of birth groups, I feel that they are specially good for first-time parents. It's like medical students. They are much more fun to have around than residents or doctors because they still have a certain eagerness and interest and curiosity. Also, they have some special issues to cover, and the same thing is true for new parents who are getting together and sharing their ignorance. Those exchanges provide comradeship and a realization that others are going through the same thing. Also, it's helpful to have someone who is experienced like you—in working out and understanding those relationships from a different standpoint—guiding the group.

Rachel: I think a birth group is still important for parents who have more than one child. I have a certain amount of anxiety about this new pregnancy. I wonder how I'm going to do it all. It would be good to talk to other mothers about what they do—it would ease my anxiety.

Alan: Now that you mention it, I can certainly see it would be valuable for us to be involved in another group like that. Maybe even a mixed one with first-timers as well as old-timers. I feel a qualitative difference between the first pregnancy and this because we focused on that one. I recall it as a magical, idyllic period.

We started going to your birth group in New York when we weren't even pregnant—until the end of the group. Rachel got pregnant just a couple of months before we left for here. The most important part of that

time was that it was a great transition in our lives. We
were negotiating our relationship to allow ourselves to
become a family.

My feelings about life are that love and romance are
the glue that allow almost impossible things to happen
between people. Because otherwise it doesn't make much
sense for people to be together, because everyone's so
different they will never get along completely. Only love
and intangibles like that keep people and families
together. The romance keeps things together while the
practical things get worked out. Now I'm less romantic
about having a baby. I can feel a rekindling of memory
of the first time. . . .

Rachel: It's fun talking about it—I now have such a
different point of view. I was in awe of it all. I'm not
looking forward to having my figure go again. The first
time it was awesome to watch it happen. This time I
know what's going to happen. I'm going to get a big
belly. But I know I'll probably get caught up in the
magic again.

Alan: I would like to see a birth group here like we had
in New York. It would force people to turn their TV sets
off and give them a chance to discuss their relationship
in front of other people and get some things resolved
that they may have been putting off. I know we had
several of those issues, though none of them stands out
in my mind clearly at this point. Those meetings
produced a lot of emotional feelings.

We've changed a lot—a group would have a very
different meaning right now—I'm sure the issues we
would be bringing up would be much different.

Rachel: At the time, though, having a baby in an
unconventional way was going against the trend. I really
felt I needed support—going to the group, reading the
books, talking to the other women to build up that
determination that I was going to do it.

Alan: There was a whole gamut of different responses in the group—even though we had similar values and attitudes. Several families from the group had their babies in the hospital, one at home, one at a birth center, for instance. We were all happy for each other and it was the right thing to do it the way we each did it. There was support for the way each couple went to the finish line.

Rachel: You never told people how they should do it. We were just told about the possibilities.

Alan: The group didn't create unrealistic pressures, or claim that everyone should have a home birth. Even though you want natural childbirth, it's possible that you may have to have a C-section. The important thing is to have a healthy baby!

Some larger patterns of response began to emerge from the interviews I collected. Several aspects were striking to me. Six years after the birth of their children, some of the men showed a tendency to minimize the needs and vulnerabilities they clearly felt during the first pregnancy. Their wives, in contrast, vividly remembered how crucial the support groups had been for them. What might be the source of the father's reluctance to acknowledge their need—a reluctance that may make it difficult for men to join a birth group in the first place? I suspect that men feel a cultural pressure to be masterful, strong and dependable in the face of their impending parenthood—an honorable impulse, but an impossible demand. This pressure makes it even more difficult for them to express the complex of feelings—ambivalence, envy, rejection—that accompanies pregnancy. In the group, men could share these taboo feelings, but later on, it seemed more difficult for them to admit how frightening and immediate these feelings had been. Other men experienced this vulnerability in ways that allowed them to make a transition to new, deeper and stronger levels of feeling. In contrast, *not one* of the women denied the need for such support groups. Men were agreeable if their wives wanted them to attend, but few felt strong personal motivation to join on their own initiative. It's my hope that a father's psychological participation during pregnancy and birth will come to be seen increasingly as a source of personal gratification for men, and will not be something that is done simply to please their partners.

Another thread that became apparent was the issue of ambivalence toward authority—in this context, the medical professionals. In some cases, parents were torn between the natural desire to be taken care of, to give up autonomy and the more socially acceptable pressure to decide for themselves and guide the birth experience. If this ambivalence is not cleared up during the pregnancy, the result can be disappointing—if not disasterously confusing during labor and delivery, with mother and doctor at odds. A birth group can help couples decide what kind of birth they *really* want, and for what reason, and then help them plan for it. For example, there should not be pressure to have a midwife if that is not what the couple truly desires—or to have a home birth. If the choice is not made with full awareness of the pros and cons, they may not be able to handle the responsibility. The important goal is to clarify the personal attitudes and desires of each couple.

Although each couple had their own individual words of praise or criticism for the place of the group in their lives, the overwhelming general impression was that it provided focus during a difficult time.

In sharing feelings and experience, the group became aware of the cultural attitudes with which they were raised—the taboos, the expectations, the limitations, the myths. Exposing these assumptions allowed them to sense the ways in which they were either continuing the same patterned responses, rebelling against them, or evolving a personal value system.

Most people remembered the birth itself much more than the pregnancy's less focused feelings, although as we met once a week for months, there were more emotions to express than we had time for. Once the pregnant period was over, it seemed that those passionate concerns of pregnancy were quickly replaced by new sets of equally compelling parenting concerns.

In subsequent groups, I acted more assertively and sought backup support from a trained therapist when needed. Working with a male partner was also extremely important for two reasons. It allowed one of us to sit back and observe while the other was involved, and it allowed couples to view us as supportive or nonsupportive parent figures—as both the good and bad mother and father. I feel that directness and honesty for the leaders and from the group leads to expansion and growth as long as it is within a caring and supportive context. Problems that seem critical and need more private time can be handled by a consulting therapist. In fact, I would recommend for each couple a private session with the leaders once every few weeks as well.

It has been reported in research on the emotional aspect of birth that those who allow themselves to confront their deepest conflicts before the birth have an easier time afterwards. We will know more as we explore further. We are only beginning to collect data on this particular family transition, and even as we do, the structure of contemporary family life is changing.

In my discussion at the onset of the group meetings, I had emphasized that we were going to be dealing with emotional issues relevant to pregnancy. It was to be an exploratory group—not a therapy group in the generally accepted sense of that word. In planning such groups, I realize that it is important to be very specific about the goals and psychological boundaries you wish to set for yourselves.

Each couple in such groups is working at a creative task, trying to be shapers of their experience, experimenting with new attitudes and behavior, making choices that might allow a more harmonious flow with the natural order of the universe—"man in nature" as opposed to "man over nature." It can be an enriching process, as Sam said:

*   *   *

We witnessed dramatic changes in the lives of each
couple, not only around the subject of birth.

However, experiencing feelings in the group was by no means a
panacea. Anne added:

Not everything was solved in the group. My own
weaknesses persisted and persist still. A couple can't
rearrange the total pattern of their lives in five months.
I spent thirty-two years becoming who I was and
learning to behave the way I do. Learning a new way
wasn't about to happen overnight. However, the group
showed us a way of approaching the experience of
pregnancy and birth—which *did* thoroughly rearrange
our lives!

Changes, transition, process. New roles, new status, new
responsibilities to confront. Yet in touch with the universalities of
the transition, everyone connected to the same source, fed by the
same wellspring. As the group shared deeply with others, as they
listened sensitively, it became apparent that we were connected.
Another's story was one's own, another's insight clarified one's
own dilemma.

These groups met in the early '70s. Since then, the medical
management of birth has changed in two directions. Technology
has developed further, and the use of techniques such as fetal
monitoring and sonography has become even more routine. At the
same time, the art of midwifery has been revived and has begun to
play an honored role in American obstetrical practice—both in
the hospital and at home births, which have become another
alternative. Consumer pressure has been responsible for making
some of these alternative choices available. However, while attitudes about midwives and fathers and the uses of medical technology may have changed, the needs of pregnant couples haven't.

The task is learning to identify conflicts that are primal and personal in comparison to those that are the more superficial, culturally influenced ones. Different types of conflicts call for different solutions.

In some cases, changes in the medical system may be necessary; in others, turning inward and exploring one's own past and present will be the solution. For many couples, a group may serve as a guiding thread to the way out of the maze.

You can *plan for* any kind of birth, keeping in mind that what actually happens may not be under the control of you or anyone else. But no matter what your feelings are about your baby's birth, it is crucial to be able to move onward from the birth experience into the new relationship with your child. Your love and care are *the* most important aspects of your baby's life.

VII

Guidelines for Starting Your Own Group

Mothering and fathering may be instinctual,
but as each change in our world further rips the
ancient web of human life, love and instinct
need a bit more help.

Marshall Klaus

There are, of course, innumerable ways to design pregnancy workshops. The characteristics and needs of the group will be the defining factors. You will need first to begin to find people for the group. Perhaps you will know another pregnant couple who is interested in working with you. Together you may come up with ideas for finding more couples for the group or you may decide to form a group with just the four of you. You can speak with your obstetrician or other doctors to get a list of potential group members. They can be contacted by phone to propose the idea. Phoning church or school offices, the hospital where you are getting prenatal care, also may be a way of contacting pregnant couples—perhaps a notice will be posted on a church bulletin board or printed in a PTA newsletter. Placing an ad in a local paper is a way of reaching many people, a few of whom may be interested. Remember, you do not need to find a lot of people—just a few more interested couples is all you'll need. Perhaps there are local bulletin boards that you know of where notices are posted—if so, this is another way of reaching out. Perhaps, a notice at stores that sell baby clothing and furniture, health food stores or local Red Cross offices, laundromats, or bookstores. You might emphasize on your notice that it is a group for first-time parents since it seems best when everyone is starting from the same emotional stage as a parent.

Childbirth education teachers are a good reference source, too, and may be of some help in forming the group. They may be able to refer members of their prepared childbirth classes to you. You may even enlist a childbirth educator to help out with the group, at times when you may wish to have a leader to direct a particular exercise. It's quite possible to just begin talking with a pregnant woman you happen to see in a café or shop! You'll soon get a sense if she might be interested in the group work you're planning and you can propose this on the spot.

It's most advisable to begin this exploration early in pregnancy, with as much of the pregnancy still to come as possible. The third month would be the very best time to begin, for then the pregnancy has become quite real to both of you, while much time still lies ahead for unfolding and exploring. Usually the class for labor and birth preparation is begun in the seventh or eighth month, so it is well to begin this very different sort of exploration and learning early on.

What is the ideal size for a pregnancy support group?

The groups should be small—eight to ten members are best. Small groups allow each person more time to participate and to be seen and heard. Also, trust and intimacy develop more easily among fewer people. If you are sensitive to allowing each person to participate in his or her way, at his or her own speed, a natural unfolding will take place. It may not even happen during the group, but later on. People unfold in different ways.

I have contacted five interested couples. We've agreed to meet once a week for four months. What do we do next?

If you feel more comfortable having a family therapist or childbirth educator to guide your group, you can contact your local family practitioner or write to the International Childbirth Education Association, P.O. Box 5852, Milwaukee, Wisconsin 53220, for the names of people in your hometown who are interested in doing this kind of prenatal counseling. Family counseling is being recognized as a vitally important service, and it may be possible to find a sponsor to fund your group. If you can arrange to have male and female coleaders, so much the better. Or, you may just decide to plunge in and do it yourselves, using this book as your guide. The success of consciousness-raising groups in the past years has taught us to value self-led groups; people involved in the same experience have a lot to offer each other. Self-led groups will develop differently from those led by a therapist or counselor—all are useful.

If you are doing it on your own, it would be wise to have a list of therapists who are available for backup support or counseling, in case issues come up for individual couples who need more time or different skills than the group can provide. Trust your heart and your intuition. Respect the fact that you know a lot about what others are feeling; you're feeling many of the same things. In this case, I'd recommend that each couple read this book prior to meeting the first night. In Chapter VIII I've written out, in some detail, exercises that I've found to be useful in my own experience as a leader. You may wish to substitute or add others. At the first meeting, you might agree to begin with the first exercise and move on at your own speed. Different couples can take turns leading the exercises, so that everyone gets a chance to participate.

I've only been able to find one other pregnant couple where both the partners are interested. Can we function effectively as a group?

Definitely. There are no limitations on what you can accomplish. More isn't necessarily better, only different. The important thing is your willingness to air your feelings and concerns.

I'm a single woman, thirty-five, who has decided to have a child on her own. How do I fit in? I desperately need a support group.

You're not alone! Your doctor or people at the local women's clinic will surely know of other women who've made decisions similar to yours, who also need the support and encouragement you are wisely seeking. As more women decide to have children on their own, there will be more demand for prenatal groups composed of partners who may simply be close friends, whether female or male. Ideally, this partner will be the person who will be helping out at the time of your baby's birth, so that you can begin to develop the kind of deep trust and intimacy that you need during the final stages of pregnancy, labor and delivery.

Do we really need to begin with a weekend session, as you recommend?

When possible, I do suggest that the group begin with a two-day session held over a weekend. It's wonderful if you can take over a friend's house in the country and spend the night, bedding down with sleeping bags and eating meals together. Such an extended period of contact at the start gives people an opportunity to get to know each other in depth. You will be less distracted. A certain psychological momentum can develop under these conditions. Bonds can be established that allow true intimacy to develop more quickly than otherwise would be possible. This process can't be rushed, and each group will have its own patterns of growth and development. It has advantages. One special bonus is getting away together, something that becomes more difficult once the baby is born. Now is the time to enjoy each other and revel in your free time.

After the weekend, if that is the way you begin, the group should agree to meet one night a week. Thereafter, if that is too often for some members' schedules, it could be every other week; however I would strongly recommend a more continuous format. Not only does a couple need the ongoing support, but there is so much to deal with that there never seems enough time for everyone.

Whether or not you can take the time for a weekend, it will be wise to start the group with a design similar to that suggested in the weekend workshop format that follows. Simply break it up into sections. Use the first morning plan for your first evening, the afternoon for your second evening, and so forth. Let the structure develop gradually so that you can create a safe, supportive climate for each other.

During this vulnerable period when you are affecting each other and your child in such profound ways, it seems important to take time to readjust, to move through the transition into parenthood gradually so that it can be a creative learning period and a source of pleasure.

You will want a warm and relaxing environment for your meetings. Rotating the meetings from house to house is one possibility. Be sure that you have the space to yourselves so that there are no interruptions. Other possibilities are church and school meeting rooms, but they tend to be impersonal and not conducive to the intimacy that needs to develop. Working outdoors tends to be distracting. A residential environment is probably best. Soft places to sit are important, as well as a rug on the floor, cushions that comfortably support pregnant bodies and a clear space somewhere with no furniture so that there is room for you to lie down during the exercise portion of the meeting. Clear away coffee tables or any furniture that creates a physical barrier between the members of the group, for it may also create psychological distance. Be aware of the environment as a supportive element for the group gathering, and embellish or empty it in whatever ways you feel will help to create an intimate ambience. Lighting will be an important factor. It should be soft and indirect and yet bright enough for everyone to see subtle facial expressions. You will need a record player and a tape recorder.

Here are some general suggestions about the group process:

Begin the group as early in the evening as possible, for there should be a definite closing time. Groups should not run late, on and on. Pregnant women become tired in the evening and do need a lot of sleep, and a too-late group won't accomplish much. Prepare the meeting room in advance and perhaps bring a vase of flowers for a special welcome.

Honor this time. Create relaxed time and quiet for this work. Take the phone off the hook if necessary. It is helpful to begin each evening with a relaxation exercise (meditation and breathing exercise). Use music to start a session if that creates calm. Follow it with another more thematic exercise or not, as you like. An initial period of relaxation and focused breathing loosens everyone up and facilitates discussion. Be sure to give directions for the exercises slowly. It's surprising how much we can experience if not rushed. Be flexible. Let the concerns of the evening determine the structure of the session, if they are urgent ones. When something powerful is happening for one person, a couple or for the group itself, scuttle the planned exercise and talk or improvise an exercise that feels right. It usually will be relevant for others. Don't push others faster than they want to go. Most of us know our own limits.

Explore; be creative. Trust your judgment. Follow the feelings that arise. Listen with your heart as well as with your mind. Useful questions for the leader to ask group members during various exercises may be: *What is happening right now for you? What are you feeling? Where do you feel it? What just happened?*

As different themes emerge, different exercises will be appropriate. Also, themes may occur in another order than I have listed them. The exact order is not important, since this is only a suggestion of progression and the dynamics of each group will differ. Basic themes will arise over and over, each time in a guise appropriate to current issues. The same exercises can be tried more than once to yield new insights. You may feel these exercises are too formal an approach, or they may appear to be mechanical and manipulative. Give them a try. I have found that they catalyze deeper levels of feelings which, when once invited, continue to reveal themselves.

You can use a variety of awareness-enhancing techniques that have been developed over the past several decades, as well as ancient Eastern ones. I improvised some myself as the group progressed. You can, too. The spectrum of techniques includes: guided fantasy, Gestalt awareness, a variety of meditation and focusing techniques, drawing and work with clay, journals, psychodrama, massage and body awareness exercises. You can use films and slide shows also.

After about an hour and a half, people will need a break, to stretch, walk around and nibble on refreshments. After fifteen minutes, the group should gather again so that the momentum of the evening is not dissipated in casual chatter and socializing.

Move gently into the sharing process. Some people are eager to share with others their innermost thoughts and feelings. Others are more private until trust has been established. Feeling coerced doesn't develop a feeling of trust. The pregnant year is a vulnerable time. Confidentiality may be important until everyone checks with his-her partner to make sure which areas of confidentiality are to be preserved for now. Surprises aren't supportive! It might be a good idea to check out points that you suspect are sensitive before they are aired in front of the whole group. As the group develops, trust will be established. At the beginning, opt for creating a safe environment.

Variations on the Basic Group

Separate Strands: A Women's Group, A Men's Group

For each parent, the strands of reevaluating one's self-image, understanding one's changing identity and confronting one's insecurities are an intrinsic part of the workshop. If women have little opportunity to express their conflicting emotions during pregnancy, men have far less. One way to encourage men to practice expressing their pregnancy-related feelings in a "safe" environment is to sometimes begin an evening by letting the men and women break up into separate groups for the first half of the evening. Then, after the break, couples can get together and in the group setting discuss what had emerged earlier.

In my experience, this variation was an important source of new information for the men and women who participated. They found that they really needed intimacy with and expressions of support from their own sex as well as from their partners. They needed to know which concerns were personal to them alone, which were common to other men or women and which issues were equally relevant to both sexes. There were charged subjects, such as sex or money, which elicited different responses depending on the gender makeup of the group. It's crucial that these differances be acknowledged by discussing them in the larger group, if a deeper understanding between couples is to be achieved. The results from one of my workshops were particularly illuminating and I include some of this material here to show you the potential insights that can be gained from this variation.

It was fascinating to see the unexpected direction taken by the women. Not babies, not personal appearance or sexuality, but work and career were the "forbidden" subjects that the women gravitated towards among themselves.

Three of the women had been working in professional careers and had become quite independent and respected in their fields. They now feared that motherhood and domesticity would force them into a restricted and dependent position. An animated discussion took place, often with all the women talking at once and then laughing at themselves. Alone with other women, they talked spontaneously and passionately, interrupting each other constantly, expressing feelings, affection and strong attitudes. With the men, however, they were more controlled and self-effacing, usually allowing their partners to take the dominant role, or even to speak for them, as if responding to an unspoken social norm.

With each other, they expressed passionate concern about their future, about the fear of losing their status as *real* people, about exchanging their present identities for anonymous ones, as they drowned in a morass of unending, repetitive maternal duties. They feared the loss of their hard-won competence in what they referred to as the *real world*. They were afraid it would suddenly vanish, convinced from what they saw around them that the privileges and satisfactions they enjoyed in their professional lives would be exchanged for a narrow world of maternal drudgery in which there was little feedback or acknowledgment for their competence and creativity. Fears of isolation were expressed. In fact, they were already beginning to feel devalued, unseen, unloved. Of course, they realized that they were gaining something intrinsically valuable by having a baby; nevertheless they were also poignantly aware of what they might be losing.

Why couldn't they talk openly with their partners about their concerns for their careers, their passion about their work and about getting ahead?

Just as nonpregnant women may find it difficult to be work-centered, independent and yet nonthreatening around men, so pregnant women, who have simply crossed a physiological bridge, find themselves in the same psychological bind. Indeed, their problem is intensified by yet another layer of cultural attitudes. In their pregnant state, they may feel a subtle but powerful social injunction to be obsessed with the welfare of their baby and the glories of impending motherhood, instead of their careers. For them, pregnancy amplifies the conflict between wanting to be "womanly" and "professional" at the same time.

Anne was the most concerned, and often had dared to confront the issue in the mixed group. This evening she was very active in the discussion, among the women.

> **Anne:** I'm on a kind of seesaw a lot of the time. Some of the time I feel really trapped. I'm afraid to share this with Sam. And I extend this to men in general. I feel that the glowing motherhood image is what I ought to be feeling and I'm afraid or reluctant—to tell the truth. When I discovered I was pregnant, I didn't tell Sam for three days.

> **Leni:** What would happen if you told the truth?

> **Anne:** My fantasy is that Sam would say, "You're going backward. I've wanted a child for so long, you've resisted for so long and now we're going back to that place. I thought you'd finally left it." Then he would dredge up all the bad stuff we would get into around having a child. Anyway, it's irrelevant because I *am* pregnant.

That theme ricocheted around the room; nearly everyone identified with it. It also incorporated other themes, like ambivalence, dependency and fears of being an incompetent mother.

> **Anne:** When I think of what is overwhelming me, I don't think it's the birth itself. It's the results of birth.

Will I be able to do it? Will I be good at it? Will I feel
that I am carrying most of the responsibility? What will
happen to Sam and me? Will I feel trapped?

Elena: I understand. I feel that in giving up "work" I'll
become a worthless person. I've swallowed the male
value system whole. I realized I felt sorry at one point
for a woman in my office who left to have a baby.

Anne was particularly concerned about the upcoming career
change in her life, since Sam was being transferred to the California branch of his company and she would be forced to leave her
excellent job as a result. Their situation demonstrated the stereo-
typical contrast between men's and women's commitments to
careers or raising families.

Anne and the others wanted to continue to develop as whole
persons, they wanted the continued respect they had earned in
their fields and the added stimulation of the male-female community they had grown used to in their daily work life. They feared
that the breadth and scope of the world in which they moved
would be diminished. Ria knew she wanted to experience that
world, too, but as yet had no taste of it and—now that she was
pregnant—worried that she might never be able to realize her
goals.

Consciousness-raising sessions in the women's movement have
clearly exposed the complexity and universality of these feelings,
and most of the women in the workshop had been involved in a
women's group in some way.

Anne: It's tough. We're going to become dependent
housewives, not earning our own keep. I don't want to be
caught in the backwater of domesticity, and yet I want
to take care of the child myself.

Another side of the coin was expressed by Rachel.

* * *

Rachel: We have an opportunity to drop out for a while and go back later. It's something men who are on the responsibility treadmill lack.

But the anxiety was there; the women felt it, and voiced it. It fed other feelings of uncertainty. I'm giving up so much to be a mother—but will I even be good at it? Am I going to be the perfect mother? Who's requiring me to be? My mother? My husband? Society? Who will I be when I'm a mother?

Amy: Several days ago, I was in a vicious mood. All of a sudden, it dawned on me that I was getting back at Don for making me pregnant. At one point, I asked him why he thought I was acting like this. He came right back and said that it was because he had impregnated me. I was amazed! It came to both of us in a flash.

Elena: I understand that. I was in a similar place. I get mad at Dick for some dumb thing and then resent the baby. I went through a phase when I wouldn't drink my four glasses of milk a day. Dick would pick up on that and keep track of my milk intake. That hit me because I began to feel that he was no longer caring about me but only was concerned about the baby.

It was an animated, intense discussion that exposed strong feelings and only the time constraints and the plan to join the men interrupted it.

The Men's Group

Fears about parenting consumed the men, too, we were to discover when we came back together, though different cultural pressures hooked them. Most of them looked forward to the pleasure of a family, but they were apprehensive as well. Although they realized that their world would be enlarged by a child in their lives, they, too, had a fear of being trapped, of becoming domesticated, of losing their "freedom." "It's scary—is it worth it?" "Will I be able to support them? How much do I want to be involved?"

Sharing the concerns with each other gave the men emotional support as it did the women. It allowed them to confront parenting issues outside the boundaries of the marriage relationship and they began to relate to each other in a more trusting way. Although their discussion centered around child care issues and the changes in self-images that would be involved, it took quite a different turn from the women's discussion.

> **Don:** Since my teaching load will be small next year, I am going to have a lot of free time. I will have the major role with the baby while Amy is going to school. I love the idea. I have fantasies of working with the baby nestled against me.
>
> **Eric:** Suppose the baby starts interfering with what you're doing?
>
> **Don:** I assume that it will interfere. But if I start out with the idea that my working hours are being cut by two-thirds anyway, I'm already ahead.

They talked about the difference in male and female roles from their vantage point.

> **Alan:** I have this idea, perhaps old-fashioned, that the baby is a woman's responsibility, her career. I don't think I'd enjoy or be able to spend that much time with the baby. . . .

Eric: Do you see yourself changing diapers? Getting up in the night? Raising the kid?

Alan: I'll approach it as a sacrificial gesture.

Fantasies reverberated around the room until Tom, as leader, focused the talk.

Eric: I'm in the same position as Don and I've sort of had reality thrown in my face. It hasn't made me negative but it just seems very real.

I don't plan to work at all next year and Ria will be working. I'll be writing my dissertation so in a sense I'll be working, but it won't be at a steady job with steady hours like now. So a lot of the responsibility of child care will be mine. I'll have to work out a work schedule with my library time, too. But, like you, Don, I've really been looking forward to this, saying I'm going to be super-father and this is a great thing for men to be getting into. Then I talk with my friend, who feels very much the same way. He's finding it all-consuming. He doesn't get too much sleep at night. He's getting up to share the feedings, too.

My friend feels he's gone through a postnatal depression as a new father . . . he's overwhelmed. My friend was saying that he thinks as men assume more responsibility they are going to be experiencing the postpartum blues, too. He sees men taking on all the downbeat feelings about role change that women have been saddled with, being confined, at home all the time with the child, losing their freedom, handling a new set of responsibilities. It hits me very personally right now!

Alan: Can you imagine anything more depressing? And yet, I think I'll get a lot of satisfaction from being with my child, from enjoying it, but not from changing diapers. I'll get it from seeing the child develop and from establishing a rapport with it. I do look forward to directing the child, you know, his likes and his dislikes, but as far as rearing the child. . . .

Eric: What do you suppose rearing really is?

Nick: Well, disciplining the child and changing his diapers—the negative aspects. . . .

Don: You know, as you were talking, I was reminded that my father was such a remote figure during my whole life. It bothered me a lot when I confronted that in psychoanalysis. For a time, I was so angry at my father when I realized what had actually happened. Maybe that's why I am leaning over backward in anticipation, saying to myself that I am going to be the best father that ever was and spend a lot of time with my child. I'm looking forward to it, and you're right, I drop out of my head all of the negative parts of it.

When the two groups merged later that evening, there was a sense of awkwardness, a little like the embarrassment we experienced at our first mixed teenage social.

Alan: Well, what did you women talk about?

Amy (laughing): You go first.

We traded impressions and insights gained from the separate discussions.

Amy: It's interesting that we women had a difficult time coming up with positive feelings and it seems as if the men did that very easily.

* * *

In a shocked tone Don said, "Positive feelings about the baby?"

It was funny to look back on that scene with perspective and see the reversal of concern that was exhibited. It was as if the women (like men in a classic stereotype) had retired separately to the library with their brandy to talk about "important things" like careers, while their partners repaired to the bedroom to discuss the children, the chores, and the responsibilities of daily existence. It was even funnier when we discovered that indeed the men had done just that—that concern with the subject of rearing children and child care had absorbed their attention.

Why was it easier for the women to "talk jobs" and the men to "talk babies" when they were in groups of their own sex? One explanation may be that expressing one's deeply felt concerns in certain areas in front of one's partner may be interpreted as threatening, competitive behavior. This is especially true when the roles within the relationship are being severely tested. It is difficult to transcend cultural stereotypes even in the *absence* of a baby, and sorting out one's new roles after the child's arrival is an even more difficult task. While trying to understand our attitudes during this period, we may give out confusing double messages: a pregnant woman may be saying nonverbally, "Stay off my turf," while actually saying, "Help me share the burden." Men, too, may feel this same ambivalence when anticipating the role of breadwinner and father.

As fathers in the group became more intimately involved in their own reactions to the pregnancy, they were able to consider their caretaking role during the pregnancy, labor and delivery from a less defensive position. They began to sense their unique and important personal roles in the enterprise of creating and caring for a baby.

Like Eric, they became more involved with fathering questions in their everyday exchanges with others. They found themselves initiating conversations about babies and child care with other men at work. It was new for them to put themselves forward in that way. Participating in the pregnant period and in the birth and child care afterward was the beginning of a lifetime commitment, and reflective of a changing cultural attitude that encourages a more equitable and involved role for fathers.

Two Is a Couple, Four Is a Group

Groups don't have to be large formal entities. They can be four friends getting together spontaneously to satisfy needs that are emerging for the first time. Many couples, unable to find the support system they wanted in their community, have designed their own. One couple I know started even before conception. Nancy and Bill had been living together for several years before they married. She had been married before and had a child from her first marriage. It was Bill's first marriage. Nancy, a nurse, was back in school getting a master's degree in psychology; Bill, an ex-lawyer, was starting a consulting business in conflict resolution. They lived in Los Angeles.

Although they had been talking about having a child of their own, she had been putting it off. She felt many of the circumstances would have to be different this time. She observed that her friends were feeling as unsupported during their pregnancies as she had felt the first time, and she knew she wanted much more than that. When her closest friend in her master's program confided that she too wanted to get pregnant, she began to reconsider.

These were to be second children for each of us, and we knew we needed more support during pregnancy than we'd had the first time. We'd each thought about having another child, and it occurred to us that if we had them together, we could establish a mutual support system— over and above that which our husbands could give us. Originally, the idea that our husbands needed support, too, never occurred to us.

* * *

Both conceived within a month of each other. They were delighted. They spoke to each other every day.

We were like two rolypoly children as our pregnancies advanced. We were ironic with each other; we could do that with each other. We could laugh at ourselves together.

The support system grew into a foursome as the wives and husbands met for dinner once a week, and the social occasions gradually turned into marathon parent-consciousness sessions. They would start at seven and each would have his or her turn to talk. Throughout the pregnancy they continued to meet once and sometimes twice a week. They found it helpful to know that the other couple was encountering the same problems and that they weren't abnormal. For the men it was especially good:

Pete and I started to get close when we discovered how much we had in common. Men have trouble talking about emotions, but we could share our desperation and hear what the other had done in the same situation.

They found the dynamics of their situations to be very similar:

We'd hear Kate and Pete working through something and say to each other, "That won't happen to us," and then—WHAM—a month later we'd be into the same emotional tangle.

They shared feelings about everything as it occurred, from social concerns to sexual intimacies, comparing experiences and reassuring each other.

The women "had been going at life fast and furiously—careers, marriage, children, travel, community involvement. Then we got slowed down—by houses, children, marriage, and our bodies, which took up all our time and energy." They had looked forward to time for reading and for writing during pregnancy. It never happened. They began to worry about their domesticity as they became entrenched in it:

Nancy: I felt worried about turning into a housewife—not relating to the world at large. I've been working in a man's world and then going to school in a man's world. I find neither accommodated to raising a family.

Bill was concerned about being able to meet Nancy's emotional needs and the demands of the future. It helped him to hear Pete talk, since Pete had been through it already.

Bill: After a while I felt drained. No matter what I did, it was never enough. I began to feel hopeless. There was only so much attention I could give to Nancy—only so much handholding and reassurance. In a tribal society there are more people around to help tend to the women. It helped to have Pete there. Once he broke down and almost cried—we could be there for each other.

Independence versus dependence was a recurrent issue for all four, often each partner needing more attention than it seemed comfortable to ask for.
Nancy said:

After the struggle to be independent and autonomous, I was so suddenly so vulnerable and dependent in every conceivable way . . . but it never came out in resentment towards the baby.

* * *

The dynamics of transitional change were difficult for each of them, often repressed in thought but then showing up in the body. Bill talked about the complications:

> Things were piling up for me. I had to move my office out of my house and make room for the baby, so my life was being interfered with in a dramatic way. I developed these painful back pains. I had images of having to be wheeled into the delivery room myself. When people say that women go through a lot of biological and psychological changes, I have to feel men do, too.

These four friends found they all needed a lot of help, since so much was going on all the time and in such intense ways. In the vacuum that existed, they designed something for themselves; they reached out for each other and created a new support system which was very positive for each of them. The best part, according to Bill, was:

> The foursome made it possible for me. I needed to know that what I was going through wasn't unique—I needed to talk to another man about my man problems, and about my woman problems to another woman besides my wife. It allowed for *all* kinds of combinations of interactions. We were not simply locked into our little system.

And to Nancy:

> Everything was allowable, sayable, nothing was forbidden when we got together. Our pregnancy was not isolated outside our lives but was woven in. This human event was part of our ongoing lives and did not separate us.

Very Large Groups

There may be times when you would like to lead just one session for a very large group, such as a Lamaze class or the PTA or a church club, or simply for people interested in becoming more aware of what goes on during pregnancy and childbirth. I have developed an exercise which seems to work well with groups as large as fifty to two hundred people, although it is also effective in ones as small as ten. It is a guided fantasy in which participants are led through the pregnancy, labor, and delivery. By choosing to play the role of father, mother, or baby in family units of three, each person senses the feelings that may be experienced during childbearing. (See Exercise No. 20, Guided Fantasy of Pregnancy and Birth, Chapter 8.) By now, hundreds of people have participated in this exercise under my direction, and many have told me immediately afterward or in later letters that the experience was extremely powerful for them.

One lovely letter arrived from an older man, a professor of education in the Southwest, who had been present at the birth of his grandchild after having attended a conference where I had led a large group through the guided fantasy. His account, partially reprinted here, is a striking example of the possibilities for growth that new attitudes toward birth offer us—as a society and as individuals.

Two years ago I attended your workshop on the rites of birth. An experience I had at role-playing the birth of a child gave me an unexpected insight into my own behavior as a father of seven children. The particular behavior in question was a form of flight during the birth of my children. For all seven children I felt a great need to get away from the pain, away from the blood, away from the birth. Sometimes I fell asleep, sometimes I had to be home to attend to the other children. The first time the labor was so interminably long that I just had to get out of the hospital for a walk. During those times (1950–1964) fathers seemed to be accessories anyhow, especially during the actual birth. The physician and medical persons did all the delivery tasks, and then the mother and baby were taken home to begin the new routine. I had become proficient at helping once all were home and I was, in my own mind, a good father. Hence the flight behavior wasn't of concern to me until the advent of a new era, that of natural childbirth and home births. (I realize, of course, that these had occurred at other times and places but had not been part of my conscious world.) I became aware of the new era through reading and visiting with younger people who were involved in the natural childbirth movement. I had liked the idea; I had intellectually accepted it. However, until I went to your workshop, I had not recognized my earlier fears and attendant flight behavior. So now the question arose in my mind, "Could I now be a father in attendance?"

As I expressed these thoughts to you at the time, I began to feel both guilt and frustration; guilt, in that I had run so many times, frustration, now that both my spouse and I are sterile and I would not be able to test my courage as a father in attendance. You were quick to suggest that a positive way out of both the guilt and the frustration was to help educate my sons so that they would not have the same fears, or at least help them be aware of their fears.

Last summer our son and daughter-in-law announced that they were expecting a baby and that they were planning a home delivery. I was delighted! My wife, the grandmother-to-be, a public health nurse who works full-time with high-risk pregnancies, was considerably less enthusiastic. However, she was outwardly very supportive, helping in any way she could to prepare for the birth.

The mother and father-to-be checked out the idea with a number of persons and they quickly found that some people were extremely fearful of, some even hostile, toward the home birth. Others were very supportive. To maintain their own positive approach to it all, they decided to tell only a few of their plans. Late in the pregnancy they checked with an obstetrician who was willing to deliver the baby at the hospital should it be necessary. That gave added assurance to them and us.

My wife and I began to plan for our vacation to coincide with the expected birth date. As a matter of fact, after talking it over with the parents-to-be, we decided it would be better to be with them after the birth rather than going for the birth only to find that the baby was late and having to return to work without seeing the baby or the birth. I was still coping with the fear of being there at the birth, even though I could *say* I wanted to be there—so the idea of going a little later was appealing. My spouse seemed to feel the same way. We kidded, however, with lots of people about going to help in the delivery.

As it turned out, we arrived two days before the baby was born and were able to stay four days afterwards.

Tuesday morning, January 3, at 12:30 A.M., our son Stan woke us, saying "Jo thinks the baby will be here soon, will you please join us?" The moment we walked into the room we could see the baby's head emerging. I watched Jo's face, Stan's hands and the baby's head, then body. Jo was obviously pushing, but there was no sign of pain on her face—when the baby made the final lunge Jo smiled in relief. The greatest miracle of all, to me, was that almost immediately after emerging from his mother, the baby began to breathe. There was no slapping, no holding by the feet (both of which I had in my mind as part of the ritual); he just began to breathe. Then he peed, then defecated, then cried. (I couldn't swear to the order of the last three.) Within seconds the baby was fondling his face on his mother's breast and shortly afterwards sucking. During all of this I did have enough presence of mind to look at my watch. It was 1:25. It had all happened in less than an hour.

The next day I began to reconstruct the experience, bringing to mind my thoughts and feelings during the birth. I had maintained my calm during the entire birth, sufficiently to observe others, to observe the plants, to remember the conversations. I was not nauseated by the blood or the afterbirth. I had wondered earlier if I would be. The notion that I had carried for many years, that pain was a necessity, was dispelled, as was the mystery of boiling water. The fact that family members, including children, were in the room during the delivery changed my vision of doctors and nurses dressed in green and white being the only appropriate witnesses of a birth. The children, four and eight, took the birth as a matter of fact. Jesse, the baby's four-year-old sister, was concerned that she also have some of her mother's attention. She was soon in her mother's arms. The eight-year-old boy said to me the next day, "Why isn't Jo up and eating at the table? She has already had her baby."

Three days later at the supper table we were still marveling at the beauty and normality of the birth. To what human efforts could we attribute the successful delivery? Both Jo and Stan had, almost from the time of conception, planned for the home birth; they had discussed every aspect of it. The fact that it was Jo's second baby gave her additional insights. They had really refused to accept negative what-if kinds of concerns from others. They didn't tell great-grandmother about their intentions because they were concerned about her excessive worry and fear. (I am still not sure how she feels about it, except that she is delighted that the baby is safely here and that Jo is also healthy.) They discussed the birth with the children and the other adult in the house, and finally they sought out a supportive physician who was willing to deliver the baby should there be complications requiring that they go to the hospital. He in turn knew of a pediatrician who was willing to examine the baby three days after birth.

Finally, and probably most importantly, Jo was truly in touch with her body, her feelings and her intuitions. She "knew" it was going to be all right. She never expressed a doubt. She also believes she would have felt, intuited, known, had a normal birth not been in the making. Furthermore, she recognizes that this is not necessarily the way to go for others.

I must say that being such an integral part of the birth, in view of my earlier fears, was one of the highlights of my life to this point. I learned so much; I felt such joy, experienced such beauty. I might put it this way: This experience at once took much of the mystery out of birth and added infinitely to the mystery of life! Or—my grandson's birth was my own rebirth.

VIII

Exercises for
Exploring the Emotions
of Pregnancy

Exercises do not do anything in themselves; they merely help to focus attention and awareness, a little like a microscope magnifying the field it examines in detail. They can be tools that allow you to move beneath your usual guises and defensive layers to deeper levels of intuition.

Just as dreams open a window for you to observe the complex strands of personal behavior patterns, so can these exercises. They enable you to practice new skills in order to change behavior, once outmoded patterns are recognized. It's a little like learning a new dance. First, you watch how it's done, then you have to start practicing moving your body differently so that you can do the new steps. Once you can handle the movements skillfully, you no longer need to focus on the individual steps and you find yourself dancing, freely and unselfconsciously.

Years of creative exploration and testing have created a wealth of material to draw on. Many of these methods have grown out of the fields of humanistic and transpersonal psychology over the past twenty years. The exercises that follow are gleaned from my years of personal experience as a group member and a leader. Others were improvised by me as the need for them arose. Still others may be found in the growing literature on alternative techniques for enchancing personal growth and self-knowledge. I have listed some that I have found to be useful (see Bibliography).

The needs and patterns of groups will vary.

Some groups may be more verbal and need methods that develop their weaker skills, i.e., nonverbal communication; others may already be comfortable with nonverbal ways of communicating and will need to practice articulating their feelings more clearly. In my experience, a structured exercise is often very helpful in understanding unexplained moods or behavior patterns and revealing deeper layers of feelings that are provoking the behavior. I have categorized the exercises in relation to specific themes of pregnancy, because some may be more helpful at certain times.

Some of the people in my groups felt exercises weren't necessary, that simply talking together was as effective in working through problems. Others loved them. One man, in particular, felt that talking to his unborn child while it was still in the womb was a profound and moving experience that affected the development of their relationship later on. That may be true. Personally, I feel these methods cut through carefully guarded defenses more quickly since we're all so skillful at using words to cover our real feelings!

Sadly, most of us have not been rewarded for showing our true feelings and have consequently learned to hide them. Most of us have learned all too well. But we are lost without the information they provide. Our emotions and feelings are checkpoints for our sense of balance and equilibrium as we respond to the world around us. Through them we sense and express love. If our hearts are closed, true meaning does not touch us.

The exercises that follow are some that may be used for either group sessions or with two couples or individually. If you plan to use them on your own at home, I might suggest that you have your partner or a friend whose voice you like make an audiotape for you of various exercises. Then you can lie down quietly and listen at leisure when you are in the mood. Ask the reader to speak slowly, allowing enough time for you to follow the directions without feeling rushed or having to strain to keep up. The point of these exercises is to move into quiet inner places. Be sure to find a relaxed time when you will not be interrupted. Dim the lights. Spend a few silent moments lying down before you even turn on the tape. Create the same time and space and peaceful ambience for yourself as you would for others. Start to learn how to be a good parent to yourself.

These exercises are simply a stimulant—a guide to creating your own designs, perhaps, for you know better than anyone what you need. Don't feel that there is anything sacred about these suggestions. Although there is experience behind them, it is important that they be personally meaningful, so feel free to adapt them to your own images and symbols if these don't fit. I want to emphasize that there is no routine way to design these groups and that this is not an infallible recipe book. Other methods may be gathered from the books listed in the Bibliography.

Follow your feelings and your intuition and be responsive to the needs of the group members.

Breathing and Relaxation Exercises

The source of our existence is our breath. Breathing in and breathing out. From our earliest time in our womb environment, a steady, uninterrupted flow of oxygen is crucial to our existence. Once born, each breath we draw initiates a miraculous set of complex occurences which cleanse, oxygenate and feed our entire system. Each breath, each inhalation and exhalation. The way we choose to breathe in turn affects our way of being—our physical and emotional tone and health. Even though this may seem obvious, we need to remind ourselves of its essential function in our lives. It seems particularly important during pregnancy and labor to be at ease with one's breathing, to understand its function in relaxing tension, in being attuned to the baby and one's partner. In letting go. In maintaining balance.

Many people control their feelings through their breathing pattern, often with shallow breathing or quick short breaths. I remember when I was little and scared, I controlled my fear by holding my breath. I still do unconsciously. If instead, I take deep, long slow breaths, wondrous things occur. The heart rate will drop twenty or twenty-five beats a minute, as will the blood pressure. As the body relaxes, the nervous system quiets. Energy begins to flow and there is a sensation of motion and emotion that may be expressed in crying or laughing or anger and in physical action provoked by the feelings that surface.

Becoming aware of our breathing patterns and habits helps us see how we take in the world around us and how we let it go. For centuries, the Yoga schools of different traditions in the East have taught breathing awareness exercises in order to relax, to quiet the chatter of thoughts and to achieve balance of the mind, body and spirit. These practices can help us to become attuned to the larger universal rhythm of which we are a part.

Spending some time alone (or with a partner) doing these breathing exercises is a positive way to begin the sensitive attunement that will be required during pregnancy and labor and in the development of family life with your baby.

Exercise 1: First Warm-up

This exercise is a good one to start off the evening, helpful in making the transition from the work day.

Lie down on the floor. Close your eyes and get as comfortable as you can, and, for a few breaths, concentrate on the air going in and out. Notice that you relax more as you breathe out and that there is a slight tension as you breathe in. Notice at the end of expiration there is a brief moment when the chest stops moving completely before it takes another breath. This is the moment of deepest relaxation and is our own internal means of momentary relaxation. Try to exaggerate the moment when your breath is all the way out, just before you take in another breath.

Now imagine that your entire body is a vessel for air and not only your lungs but your whole body fills and empties with each breath. . . . Imagine the air filling up your whole body, all the way down to your toes. You can actually begin to feel your whole body breathing and expanding as it takes a breath and then you let go of that breath.

Imagine the breath going all the way down to the toes and that you breathe out through your feet, leaving them relaxed, emptying them of their tension. Concentrate on that end point of breathing, filling your legs each time with the new breath and emptying them out. Now fill your legs up to the thighs, feeling your legs expand and contract. Now let the breath go to your toes, your groin and now the lower back. Feel the muscles soften at the end of each breath. . . .

Now out the chest, the lower abdomen, feel the stomach muscles soften, now the chest itself, filling the whole body with air and letting it all out. No force is necessary. The air can move itself.

Now the shoulders . . . let them fill and empty. Let them feel soft and droopy. And the arms. Now the neck . . . let the neck and the rest of your body fill, empty, soften. And your head . . . feel your head getting lighter and more relaxed. . . . Continue to breathe gently and when you are ready, open your eyes.

Now your arms and hands. . . . You may notice a sensation of flowing as your body fills and then empties, now your head and scalp and your facial muscles. . . . Notice how heavy your jaw is. . . . Let your face fill with air. . . . For a few breaths, let your whole body fill and empty, the air moving up and down, feel it all over and then whenever you're ready, you can let your eyes open slowly, but when you do, allow them to open and look ahead with an unfocused gaze for a few moments while your mind relaxes and readjusts.

Breathe naturally and sense the cleansed feelings in your body.

Exercise 2: Second Warm-up

Couple by couple, lie down in the center of the room. Heads facing out, in the wide part of the circle, feet in the middle, all the feet in the middle touching.

Focus on your breathing and start to let go. Continue to breathe naturally and gently. Put your arms at your sides and let go of the tension in your head, first of all. Let your head sink right into the floor, let it go . . . lose its weight.

Starting with your brow, begin to relax, wrinkle it and unwrinkle it for a minute, so that it's very relaxed. Squeeze your eyes, then let them go. Tighten up your nose, wiggle it around and let it go. Be aware of your cheeks, and relax them . . . and your mouth, tense it and let go. Tense the muscles of your chin, and your jaw, and then let them go.

And now your shoulders, let them sink right into the floor, first your left one and then your right one and now your back. Tense it, if it helps, before you relax it. Feel the back go into the floor. Let your waist go into the floor, relax it. And now your stomach, tense those muscles, let them go. And your pelvis, tense the muscles very, very tight, and then let them go.

Now your thighs, tense them, very tight, and let go. And now, the lower part of your legs, your calves, tense them, let go. Now your arms, first the upper part of your arms, tense the muscles and relax them. And the lower part of your arms, tense and let them go.

Focus your hands, wiggle your fingers, and let them melt into the floor. And now, lie still, relaxed, let your body sink into the floor and the earth below it . . . let your mind go. . . .

Exercise 3: The Unfolding Rose

This exercise is adapted from a psychosynthesis technique and will be useful throughout the pregnancy, as well as during labor. The symbol of the flower has been used in both East and

West to denote the inner self; the spiritual self. In China, it has been the "Golden Flower"; in India and Tibet, the lotus; in Europe and Persia, the rose. The flower is rooted in the earth, and nourished by the water and the sun. Its development from bud to fully open bloom parallels the pregnancy process.

Lie down in a comfortable place or sit in a chair. Close your eyes. Vizualize a tightly closed green rosebud. Then move back along the stem until you come to the main branch. Imagine the whole bush with all its leaves and branches and buds, with its roots growing out of the earth.

Then move slowly back to the bud. Imagine the rose opening very slowly, revealing the tip of a delicate pink flower. Watch the flower slowly unfold.

Become the rose. The sun is shining on you. Its warmth hastens your blossoming. Gentle dew covers the surface of your petals and the sun is reflected through the droplets of water. The air caresses you. A gentle breeze ruffles the surface of your petals. The sun fills you with its energy and you open still further. Your sweet, delicate scent is released. You continue to unfold, expanding until you are completely open—in full bloom.

Exercise 4: Sensing Your Environment

Get comfortable, close your eyes, take a few very deep breaths. As you inhale and exhale, slowly follow your breath through your body and out again. Concentrate your mind on your breath. Be aware of your feelings and sensations but don't judge your thoughts, simply allow them to be there and then let go of those feelings and thoughts.

Sense your stillness and then, as you lift your hand, feel how everything changes. Lie still again and then move your foot. Again sense what happens in your body. Is it only movement? Is there sound? Is there a shift of color or form in your mind's eye? Wiggle your waist. What happens?

Touch your clothing and feel the differences of textures. Do different colors feel different? Touch your skin. How does that feel? Focus on the scent in the room. What does it smell like? Have you been aware of it right along? Does it remind you of anything?

Focus again on your breathing. Be aware of the movement it generates in your body. Be aware of your breath and energy moving out of your body into the room and mingling with the flow of others' energy and becoming part of the sound, smell and movement of the room.

When you are ready, open your eyes slowly and look around the room. Be sensitive to color, form, movement, texture, smell and to the feelings they provoke in you. Continue to use this awareness as you interact with others to understand how these perceptions affect you in the course of your day.

Exercise 5: Getting Acquainted

As the group sits in a circle, each person can introduce him or herself briefly, saying whatever each feels important to share. After each person has spoken, you can spend a few minutes learning each other's names. Everyone in turn says their name and turns to the next person, who repeats the preceding names and then says his or her name. For example: "You're John. You're Susan. You're Bill. I'm Leni. . . ." until the last person in the circle has repeated all the names of the people that have preceded him. It sounds difficult and maybe embarrassing, but it works well, not only for learning everyone's name, but also for getting people laughing and in a lighter, relaxed state.

Exercise 6: Guided Fantasy—Watching Thoughts

Close your eyes and get into a comfortable position. . . . Be aware of whatever thoughts, words, or images are going through your mind.

Imagine that you are in a large room, with two ample doorways on opposite walls. Imagine that your thoughts and images come into this room through one doorway and then go out of the room through the other doorway. Simply watch your thoughts as they move into the room. Let them remain in this room for a while and then move out again. Don't get attached to them. Let them exist apart from you. Simply view them from afar. Observe them. . . .

What are they like? What do they do while they're in the room? How do they come in? How do they go out? Do they rush in and out? Or do they settle into the room gradually so that you can see them separately and clearly?

What happens if you close the exit door? Now open it again. . . . Now close the entrance door and notice what happens. . . . Open it again. . . . Now close both doors and notice what happens. . . . Open them up again. . . . Now close both doors at once and collect a few of your thoughts to bring them back to this room with us. . . .

When you have gathered them, collected them, examine them as carefully as you can. . . . What are they like? How do they act? What do they do now? How do you feel towards these thoughts and how do they respond to you? Talk to them and let them answer you. . . . Now become your thoughts and continue the dialogue. . . . Let all the thoughts bump into each other. . . . Let one emerge . . . and hold it. . . . Look at it from all sides. . . . When you are ready, open your eyes. And share what's been happening.

Exercise 7: Massage Circles

An Opening Exercise for the Beginning of the Evening

The group sits on the floor in a circle, alternating men and women, with new partners on either side. All join hands and close eyes, sitting quietly as they are led through a relaxation exercise. After about five minutes, each person does a half turn to the left and is sitting behind another. Each person massages the head, neck and back of the person in front of them. After about seven minutes, everyone reverses and massages the person who has just massaged them.

Exercise 8: Group Rock

An exercise that expresses affection and caring and also evokes trusting feelings from the person who is being rocked. It's an especially good exercise for men but nurturing for everyone.

The person to be rocked lies on the floor, and closes his-her eyes. Each member of the group kneels down and puts their hands under a section of the body that they will lift—one person takes the head, another one a shoulder, another the waist, another the hips, another the lower leg, another the feet and so forth, distributing the weight evenly among the group. Then the group lifts the person slowly in a horizontal position as high as they can and rocks them gently back and forth slowly and rhythmically as long as it is comfortable—taking quite a bit of time. When they are ready, they gradually lower the person to the floor, chanting, singing or humming in accompaniment to the movement. The rocked person should lie quietly afterward, absorbing the feelings. This can be done for any group member who requests it, or one member might ask another if he-she would like to be rocked during a stressful evening.

Exercise 9: Trust Circle

One person stands in the center of a circle formed by the group of about six to eight members. The person in the middle closes his-her eyes and relaxes completely and allows him-herself to be passed around the circle from person to person. If the person is heavy, two people may hold the person as they are being passed.

He-she may be turned when passed or held for a moment and hugged. The important thing is to relax and allow oneself to be supported by the group.

Exercise 10: Blind Walk

Partners take turns closing their eyes and allow themselves to be guided wordlessly through the space, trusting that their partners will take care of them. They may lead each other up or downstairs, or sit their partners down, and guide them through different sound, smell and touch experiences—either outside or inside.

This sequence can be followed by a walk with another partner, also.

Exercise 11: I Need, I Want

Sit opposite your partner, looking at each other directly. Try to maintain eye contact throughout the exercise. If you find you are avoiding holding your partner's gaze, stop for a minute and be aware of the feelings you have when you begin to withdraw.

Each of you take a turn listing all the things you need. Start each sentence with "I need." Your partner will write your list as you state your needs. Get them all out . . . take about five minutes. . . . When you have exhausted them, start again and exchange "I need" with "I want." Try to consider which are essential to you and which can be eliminated. You may feel that having some emotional needs satisfied seems as important as food and water. That may be so for you . . . just try to be discriminating about your unique needs. Do the same with "I want."

After you have each had your turn, discuss what you felt about your experience throughout this exercise and about your reaction to your partner's needs and wants. What did you discover?

Exercise 12:

Try the same exercise with the following words: I Have to, I Choose to.

Exercise 13:

I Can't, I Won't.

Exercise 14: Expressing Ambivalence

This exercise can be done in two different ways. 1. Each person chooses a partner other than his/her own, either a man or a woman. 2. Each partner should write a list following the instructions below:

Take a few minutes to think of all the reasons why you would like to have a baby and then either tell your partner or write your list. If you are working with a partner, the listener should simply receive what is being said, without responding. After one is finished, the other takes a turn.

When both have completed their thoughts, think of all the reasons why you *don't* want to have a baby. And listen to each other again.

After completing this part of the exercise, the whole group can share feelings with each other and couples can either break off in pairs afterward for further discussion or continue to share with the group.

There may be some deep and troubling feelings released that require further work. Ambivalence is an important issue to deal with.

Exercise 15: Inside the Womb

This is an exercise that gives you a sense of what it may feel like to be inside the womb.

Form groups of four. Stand close together in a circle with arms around each other. Be still for a few minutes with your eyes closed. Become aware of your breathing, of the rise and fall of your chest. . . . Expand your awareness to include those standing beside you and sense the rhythm of their breathing. . . .

Open your eyes and with a soft unfocused gaze and, without words, take in all the members of the group . . . the person opposite you   . . and those beside you. . . .

One by one, in turn, bend from the waist and put your head between the bodies of your group, first at the level of their hearts and then at the level of their abdomens. The other three, with arms still around each other, form an enfolding circle. Remain still and focus on creating a synchronized feeling among the group members.

It is helpful to keep your eyes closed throughout the experience. When you are in the center, take as long as you like to have the experience of being held.

Exercise 16: Meditating with the Baby

This is an exercise designed to focus on the links between mother and father and unborn baby as a threesome. Each partner in a couple sits facing each other, joins hands and closes their eyes as you begin with a relaxation exercise.

Then with eyes still closed, and hands joined, meditate on yourself as a family, on yourself as partners, as a mother or father. Be aware of the life growing inside the womb. Sense your baby. Get in touch with your individual breathing and then feel the movement between you as a couple. Allow your breath to flow from one to the other and then to the baby until you feel you are in rhythm with each other. Visualize the baby's environment inside the womb and imagine what the baby might be experiencing. Consider its sense of you and of the outside world and what you might be communicating to the baby. Think about your feelings as a mother and as a father and stay in touch with yourselves as a threesome. . . .

When you are ready, open your eyes. Take a few minutes in silence and then write a conversation with the baby.

Exercise 17: One Becoming Two Becoming Three

Get into a comfortable position. Close your eyes. . . .

Think about your week . . . how has it been? Think about your pregnant body . . . the baby inside you . . . your impending motherhood . . . . And fathers, think about your baby inside your partner's womb and about your own body and your impending fatherhood.

Is there anything that's been special about this week? Has anything been particularly meaningful? Was it related to your pregnant state? Any new or unfamiliar feelings? Either in your body or your emotions? How has it been for you as a couple this week? Is there a particular way in which you have thought about each other this week? Any special way you have interacted? Have you had any thoughts or fantasies about the way it will be when you become three instead of two? Even fleeting thoughts should be paid attention to.

Have you had any dreams this week? Take a minute to recall them. Maybe one will even spring to mind that has been forgotten.

With your eyes still closed, each couple join hands and rest your two hands over the womb. Snuggle closer to each other if that feels better. . . . Without sharing it right now with each other, each of you become aware of the baby and have a conversation or communicate in whatever personal way feels right.

With eyes still closed, start to share this experience and the happenings of the week, and the feelings you are now having.

This exercise can be used throughout the pregnancy.

Exercise 18: Birth Meditation and Drawing Exercise

Lie on the floor next to your partner and form a group wheel—a mandala, with the hands touching in the center of the wheel. Close your eyes. Fathers, place your hands over the womb, over the baby. Mothers, place your hand on your partner's hand. . . . Become aware of your breathing. Gently, breathe in and out, slowly . . . in and out . . . breathe in rhythm with each other and be aware of the baby's rhythms. Inhale . . . exhale . . . deep breaths. Fill your lungs and let the breath empty completely.

Visualize a ball of energy—a ball of light—in the middle of your forehead and hold it there. . . . Now start that ball of energy moving clockwise in a spiral around inside your head, moving downward, circling your throat and around inside your shoulders, then around into your heart. . . . Then let it circle around your heart again and around the arm that is placed on the womb. . . . The energy ball spiraling around your arm . . . into your hand . . . the hand that is connected to each other and to the baby. Let it come to rest there . . . the two balls of energy merging. . . . Remain quietly as long as it feels comfortable, perhaps three minutes.

Now gather your own energy ball again and spiral it back through and up around your heart, circling your shoulders . . . your throat and back of the middle of your forehead. . . . Let it fade slowly away.

When you are ready, open your eyes and get comfortable. Sit up. Take one piece of paper and share a box of crayons and draw together as a couple anything you want but be sure to include the baby in the picture. Use color, shape and images to express the feelings evoked. After you are finished, share with each other: How did it feel? Was it cooperative? How much space did each take up? How do you like your drawing? Then share, if you like, with the whole group.

Exercise 19: Nameless Child

Lie down. Close your eyes. After a relaxation exercise, listen to these words and move with them.

There is a mountain of gold. When the sun's rays strike it, it is irritating to look at. It is surrounded by red, green, orange, purple and pink clouds, wafted gently by the wind. Around the mountain fly thousands of copper-winged birds with silver heads and iron beaks. A ruby sun rises in the east and a crystal moon sets in the west. The whole earth is covered with pearl-dust snow. Suddenly, a luminous child without a name comes into being.

> The golden mountain is dignified,
> The sunlight is blazing red,
> Dreamlike clouds of many colors float across the sky.
> In the place where metal birds croak,
> The instantaneously born child can find no name.

Because he has no father, the child has no family line. He has never tasted milk because he has no mother. He has no one to play with because he has neither brother nor sister. Having no house to live in, he has no crib. Since he has no nanny, he has never cried. There is no civilization, so he has no toys. Since there is no point of reference, he has never found a self. He has never heard spoken language, so he has never experienced fear.

He walks in every direction, but does not come across anything. He sits down slowly on the ground. Nothing happens. The colorful world seems sometimes to exist and sometimes not. He gathers a handful of pearl-dust and slowly lets it trickle through his fingers. He gathers another handful and slowly takes it into his mouth. Hearing the pearl dust crunch between his teeth, he gazes at the ruby sun setting and the crystal moon rising. Suddenly, there's a whole galaxy of stars and he lies on his back to admire their patterns. He falls into a deep sleep, but has no dreams.

The child's world has no beginning or end.
To him, colors are neither beautiful nor ugly.
He has no preconceived notion of birth and death.

The golden mountain is solid and unchanging,
The ruby sun is all-pervading,
The crystal moon watches over millions of stars,
The child exists without preconceptions.
Chogyam Trungpa,
Dharmas Without Blame

Become the baby curled and floating in the womb. Surround yourself with these sounds, as if nothing else exists.
Afterward discuss your experience as a group.

Exercise 20: Guided Fantasy of Pregnancy and Birth

The group will form families of three and each one decide which role you would like to play. There should be a mother, father and a baby (a fetus) in this experience of pregnancy and birth. You can choose to play whatever part you wish and do some role reversing so that men can have the sense of being mothers, women of being fathers and those who choose to be babies can be whatever gender you wish. If there are more people than a three-person family accommodates, expand it into foursomes and have twins in some families.

When you have chosen your families, find a roomy place on the floor where your family can stretch out and lie down close to each other, holding hands or being in contact with each other in a way that feels comfortable. If you like you can have music in the background; Dr. Hajime Murooka's "Lullaby from the Womb" (Mother's Heartbeat—and Sounds from the Body Arteries), or Michael Jean Jarre's "Oxygen" are good ones.

Get comfortable . . . relax as fully as you can, using one of the earlier relaxation exercises.

Mothers, enfold the babies in a position that will be comfortable for a period of time. Find a position that allows the baby to feel in close body contact to you, enclosed and symbiotic. Fathers, stay close, although you may be more active in your positions and will probably move around more. Find a position that is in relationship to the mother and baby. And babies, curl up comfortably with your mother so you feel enfolded . . . in the womb of the mother.

Now the baby begins to focus on this experience and parents also will focus on this experience, trying to create it as an ideal experience for all of you—to design your own emotional birth environment—you the baby and you the mother and father, collectively creating a positive birth environment inside and outside the womb right here.

Imagine that conception has taken place—that the fertilized egg has begun to divide, splitting first into two cells, then into four. After a week, it has become a ball of cells. The baby is growing rapidly. Mothers don't know they are pregnant as yet.

Babies, sense yourselves as tiny fetuses attached to the wall of the womb, growing and expanding. And talk to your parents for a few moments about what is happening for you as you are becoming. . . . Focus on the environment in which you are living and on your parents beyond that environment. Sense the feelings that you are being imbued with and that you want to carry along—the qualities that you are sensing from your mother and father. Tell them out loud now about your sense of yourself coming to life as a combination of these two parents. Tell them about the weaknesses and the strengths that are forming you, the feminine side, the masculine side—all that you sense. With your eyes still closed, tell them what you are feeling.

Parents, don't answer your baby or get involved in conversation just now, simply listen. Let the baby experience the wonder of its beginning. When the baby is finished talking, parents can talk to each other about the pregnancy. Mothers, you have just learned that you are pregnant. Start to talk about what that means to you. Fathers, begin to respond about the way you feel and what it means to you, about your excitement, your fears, your needs, and, perhaps, even your ambivalence. Whatever you are experiencing. Babies, just listen without being involved in your parents' conversation.

Babies, you are now three months old. Inside the womb, you are learning what it is like to live between these two people. You are beginning to sense when your needs aren't being fully met and when they are. Babies, tell your parents what might make you feel totally secure and loved by your parents. And then, parents, try to accommodate the needs that your baby has expressed to you— each in your own way.

Babies, you are now six months old. Mothers, you have felt the flutterings of life for more than a month. The baby is a reality. Parents, what are you feeling? Are you able to ask for what you need? Do you know what you need from each other or others? What aren't you getting? Tell each other now what is happening for you.

Babies, simply listen to your parents' conversation without interacting with them and sense the mood and the quality of their relationship. You are quite active now. You have found your fingers and are even sucking them; you sip the fluids in the womb; you hear sounds in your mother's body and from outside her body, many vibrations. . . . After your parents are finished talking to each other, tell them what you are experiencing in the womb, what your environment is like and how their relationship affects you. Also what you would like . . . to be held more closely, perhaps to have more relaxed time together? Whatever.

Parents, be very sensitive and aware of your baby's needs as you sense them, and of your own needs, too. Tell the baby how you feel about its presence. What your hopes and expectations are. And your fears.

Fathers, how are you feeling? Isolated or involved? Will you share with the mother and the baby? Try to work out something that feels better.

We are now about eight months into pregnancy. The birth is drawing near. The baby is getting quite heavy now. It's a little harder to reach mother, physically. Her shape has changed a lot. Would you share some of the problems about that with each other and the baby? Mother, are you feeling very sexy? Would you share your thoughts and feelings about that? Father, are you feeling turned on by mother at this stage? What's interfering for you? Talk about it together.

Babies, how are you feeling about your environment? Is it getting crowded? Are you impatient? Do you move around a lot—or respond to the life around you? How? Tell your parents your feelings?

As a unit, as a family, try to meet everyone's individual needs. See if that is possible as you are near the ninth month—the end of the pregnancy. Mother, how are you doing with all your needs? What are they? Can father help you in any way? Could you speak to the baby about it? What are your feelings now as you are about to separate from your baby? In the next few minutes, tell each other what is happening for each of you.

Tomorrow is the day the baby will be born. Parents, talk to each other about what your needs are for the birth. Baby, begin to fantasize the environment in which you would like to be born. I want you to begin to construct in your mind what you each need—in terms of environment—people and physical space, in terms of the colors or light or darkness, in terms of sound and textures and temperature. Babies, decide what would make you feel welcome in the world. Let it take shape in your mind. Parents, tell each other what you need and envision and then baby, share with them what you need to make you feel nurtured and welcomed.

The three of you together share out loud what the ideal environment should be and what you want.

Are you feeling anxious or expectant or strong? What are you feeling?

It is beginning—the mother and baby know it is time for the baby to be born. The baby begins its movement through the birth canal and each of you plays your part in a way that allows this birth to be joyful. Stay in touch with each other as the birth occurs. Continue to tell each other what you need—the baby, mother, father—as the birth progresses.

Welcome the baby when it is born. Snuggle it, cuddle it, caress it.

Babies, continue to share what you need from your parents and the environment, what you sense you need to have around you. Will the mother share what she needs, after this ordeal or this joyous experience? Will the father remain in contact and assess his needs . . . what he senses he can give or not give . . . what he senses is needed from him?

Slowly begin to resettle yourselves comfortably as a family and talk to each about this experience. Stay together, in close contact with each other as you talk a few minutes.

Then share as a large group and tell how it went.

Exercise 21: Drawing the Body

Each person lies down on a life-sized piece of paper (a roll of wrapping paper is good) while another traces around his-her body shape. Each person then takes his-her paper image and fills in the inside space with a colored version of feelings, organs, bones, circulatory systems, emotions, whatever they feel is inside. After everyone is finished, after about twenty to thirty minutes, each person explains his-her picture to the others and gets feedback from the group.

Exercise 22: Who Am I?

Each of us embodies so many different aspects that it is helpful to set down all of the roles and qualities that are part of our lives. It will give you an enriched sense of how you view yourself and how you order those roles and qualities. You can see how the labels of others affect your sense of your own unique perceptions of yourself. You can also sense the ways those role boundaries may inhibit growth and development of a fuller self.

Choose a partner and, in turn, each of you list aloud the answers to the question, "Who Am I?" while your partner writes down your list. When you have exhausted all the "I am's" you can possibly think of, have your partner read them aloud. Then do the same for your partner. After both of you have completed your lists, take a few minutes to discuss what you have felt about the list you each generated. They will probably start with "I am a woman," "I am an American," "I am a daughter," and move into more unique aspects.

Follow this part of the exercise with a list of the qualities you feel you have, both the ones you're pleased with and perhaps some that get in your way: "I am generous," "I am shy," "I am self-disciplined. . . ."

You might go on to some more imaginative ways in which you envision yourself: "I am a fast-moving river," "I am a majestic mountain," "I am a knife that cuts clean," "I am an elf."

Exercise 23: I Am a House

Imagine you are a house. Describe the house. Walk around the outside of the house. Observe its color and shape. Is it open or closed? Describe the walls and windows. Of what material are they made? What is its setting? Is it isolated or set among other houses or. . . . How does it look?

How many entrances does it have? Notice the shapes of the doors. Describe them. Open the door, walk in, walk through the space and observe it in detail. Then describe it. Is it full or empty? What is its decoration? Does it have an attic or cellar? Does one or the other evoke feelings? Move through all its spaces. Touch it, smell it, sense the ambience. Are there people other than yourself in it? Are there changes you would like to make? People you would like to bring in? What are the colors? What are the shapes? Which rooms are favorites? Why? Which do you live in?

The state of my house seems to reflect the state of my mind and my emotions right now.

This exercise will probably evoke different images each time you do it. That is one of its advantages. It is also one you can do alone, as well as with others. Relax, get comfortable. Listen to a recording of the exercise, record or write your response.

Exercise 24: Family Recollections

1. What did your parents, aunts, uncles, sisters, brothers, cousins, tell you about your birth? What did you feel about what you were told?
2. What story did your parents tell you about how you were named? What did you feel about this?
Be your parents describing these things to you, via role playing. Were there any "don't be you" injunctions, like: "You almost killed me when I had you," "I suffered a lot," etc?

Exercise 25: Naming

Were you named after someone? If so, were you expected to replace someone or adopt their personalities? Was your name masculine or feminine? What qualities do you associate with your name?—first, middle, surname. What qualities did they associate with your name? Have you adopted those qualities? Do you like your name? Have you always?

Discuss naming the baby after one or the other of you. What does a name mean? Does a child become its name? What family pressures are involved? Societal pressures? What are the implications of creating an individual's identity? What was your experience with your own name? Were you named after someone? Did you want to change your name? What was the tradition you were to carry on?

Exercise 26: Childhood Attitudes

Start with a relaxation exercise as you lie in a circle with your heads meeting in the middle and your feet pointed out to the edge of the circle you have formed.

Then, with your eyes still closed, move back through time and sense yourself as a young child—at six, seven, eight or so. Recall your mother and father and your family setting. What did you know about pregnancy and birth? Did you have a younger sibling? What was said to you specifically about birth, about where babies came from? Did someone else talk about birth to you? What filters through? Take as much time as you need to reexperience those feelings and then when you are ready, open your eyes and while you are still lying in the circle, begin to share your recollections.

Exercise 27: Interviewing Your Mother and Father

During pregnancy, it can be very useful to spend some time talking to your mother about her recollections of her labor and your birth. Although it is usually not a subject that we discuss with our mothers since it is often a taboo subject in some families about which we couldn't ask or discuss, nevertheless, you will probably be surprised, as will she, by how fresh the memory is. Very often birth patterns are repeated from generation to generation, so it would be important to be aware of what preceded your experience so that you might avoid some unconscious programming.

You might propose the idea to your mother ahead of time so that she can begin to think about it and the memories can be stirred. Some women may be reluctant to recall difficult, lonely or painful times, so be sensitive to what your mother is feeling. She may need reassurance from you about why you are asking after all these years, so broach the subject with care. She'll probably be delighted to re-remember for her own sake.

Maybe it will be a monologue or perhaps a dialogue. It might be good to have a few definite things that you want to know in case you adapt an interview style. The group might discuss together what you would like to ask.

You might want to ask:

- What her pregnancy was like;
- What kind of medical care she received when pregnant;
- Whether she had any preparation for labor;
- What your father's attitude was;
- What her recollection was of the environment of birth;
- What her labor was like and who was with her;
- Her memory of the birth;
- What happened right after and in the weeks that followed;
- Were you nursed? Why yes or no.

You might tape the conversation or write down what happens. It's very helpful to do so. It's surprising how much goes by when you don't record things. And it's often informative to listen to changes of tone of voice and abrupt shifts in conversation after you absorb the content. They all have their own meaning.

One way you might bring the interviews back into the group would be to simply have the whole group report their stories back one evening and share feelings about what you learned. Another way would be to meet in two groups for part of the evening. One for the men and one for the women. It is often a good way to heighten intimacy beyond the couple. Different things may be brought out in this way.

Both groups may be able to discuss sensitive issues they find difficult to mention in the full group. Often questions of sexuality are more easily explored at the beginning in an all-men or all-women group and certainly the sexuality of pregnancy is a ripe area to be explored. This might be a good opportunity to begin discussions that can later be shared in the full group.

Follow a similar procedure with your father or other members of your family.

Exercise 28: Keeping a Journal

Discussion about keeping a journal. What might it include?

- Feelings on awakening and at the end of the day;
- Dreams, fantasies, body sensations;
- Feelings, thoughts at different points of the day;
- Feelings about the changes in your life now and in the future;
- Recording important happenings in the day;
- Drawing, writing poetry, and/or stream of consciousness writing.

Beginning the journal:

- Write a brief entry for last week.
- Write a brief entry for today.
- Those who would like to can read their entries to the group.

Exercise: 29 Crossroads in the Journey— Stepping-stones

This is an exercise I learned from Ira Progoff's *At a Journal Workshop*, one of the methods I explored in the course of my own journey. (Following the direction of this book can be a rich and fruitful method in itself for those to whom journals appeal.)

With paper and pencil in hand, take a few minutes to relax. Become still. Focus on your breathing. Empty your mind. When you feel quiet, begin to reflect on important events in your life that led you to this moment. You can reach back as far as you like. To your birth, if that feels right. Simply allow images of people, places, events, feelings to arise without judging them. You will be drawing out particular strands of your unique tapestry. Move back through time—your life—and select ten or twelve threads that connect you to this pregnant moment.

After ten or fifteen minutes of writing, the group can share their stories.

Exercise 30: A Game of Word Association

Write out as many similes as you can dream up for each of the following words and then add some words of your own:

Birth, a mother, a father, a baby, an environment for birth, breasts, blood, a doctor, a nurse. . . . Example: Birth is like the heavens shaking.

Create as many spontaneous images as you can—funny ones, whimsical, logical and illogical ones.

When you have a list of about eight to ten for each, read them aloud couple by couple. It's intriguing to see the overlaps and the differences and the connections you yourself have made.

Another version of this exercise can be to simply free-associate to these words, writing down your quick responses: blood, sex, breasts, pain, pregnancy. . . .

Exercise 31: Becoming Your Mother and Father

Close your eyes and go back to your youth. Choose an age that was important to you, around ten, eleven, or twelve. Visualize your mother. What does she look like? What is she wearing? How does she walk? What is the tone of her voice? When you feel you have a strong sense of her, open your eyes and stand up. Begin to circulate around the room taking on the role of your mother. Become her. Walk the way you remember her walking, talk the way she talked. Act her part as well as you can. Move among the other "mothers" and talk to each other about pregnancy and birth. You can imagine that each of you is pregnant or that you have just given birth. You will find that it is quite easy to take on her physical and emotional characteristics.

After about five to ten minutes, switch and become your father. Take time to close your eyes again and get into visualizing him as you did your mother before you begin to act the role.

Exercise 32: Father's Fantasy of Being Pregnant

The men in the group sit in a circle in the center of the room and imagine that *they* are the pregnant mothers. Stuffing a small pillow under their shirts can help the role reversal.

Close your eyes. Breathe gently and naturally, allowing your breath to rise and fall without needing to change it. Feel your belly with your hands. Feel the roundness of it, the firmness of it, feel the pressure of the uterus against your chest and the bulge resting on your lap. Your belly has been growing gradually for the past months—you are seven months pregnant. You are feeling full and ripe. The baby is moving around inside you, kicking, turning, making its presence felt. Share with the other "mothers" what you are feeling.

Exercise 33: Couple Meditation—Getting Your Needs Met

Close your eyes. Get comfortable. Sit opposite each other. Empty your mind of thoughts as best you can. Focus your attention on your breathing as your chest moves in and out, and as your abdomen rises and falls, feel your breathing deepen. When you feel still, join hands with your spouse, hold each other gently and, with eyes still closed, focus your attention on each other. . . . Is there something you would like to ask for—more attention? More privacy? Less of something?

When you are ready, open your eyes and continue to look at each other without exchanging words. When you have had enough quiet time, share with each other verbally what you would like from the other. . . . Each of you take five minutes or so, without interruption from your partner.

When you are finished with this part of the exercise, share with each other the feelings and thoughts that were occurring as the other one spoke. Stay in touch with your body reactions throughout, making note of how you feel and where you feel it. Share with the whole group when you are finished exchanging with each other, if you care to.

Exercise 34: Giving and Taking

The group sits on the floor in a circle. One person who has trouble receiving sits in the center of the circle and sits with his-her eyes closed. Each person gives to them, in turn, nonverbally, without words. The person in the center of the circle has his-her eyes closed. Another may take his-her place. Afterward, everyone shares their feelings. Often, after a couple has ventilated angry feelings towards each other, we form a "love" circle with the couple standing in the middle and the others surrounding them closely in a group hug.

Exercise 35: I Appreciate, I Resent

"I Appreciate" is a lovely and important follow-up for "I Resent" and might be combined as an exercise:

Each member of a couple sits opposite each other and, one at a time, taking about five minutes each, tells the other what they resent about the other's behavior.

I appreciate follows the same procedure, and partners tell each other in turn what they appreciate about the other.

Exercise 36: A Fantasy Shopping Trip— Giving and Taking

Close your eyes and get comfortable. . . . Imagine you are wandering down a street, looking in the shop windows, trying to find a wonderful gift for your partner. Choose a place anywhere in the world . . . be free and fanciful about your choices. Imagine the time of day . . . and the weather . . . and continue walking in the scene you are creating.

Visualize your partner, think about what he or she likes, what would please him or her. . . . When you find the place that carries the sort of gift you might like to choose, open the door, if there is a door. Walk inside, look around and choose a gift that is very particular for your partner. It may be an object, a thing, or it may be a quality that embodies your feeling. The gift will express some of the feelings that you have about him or her. Choose one gift or maybe two. Perhaps you will have to go to another shop for the second gift. When you have your gift, open your eyes. As a group, go around the circle and give your partner your imaginary gift and tell him or her what it means to you.

Exercise 37: Asking—Receiving

One father in the group who had an easy time giving and a difficult time receiving was asked to go around the room and ask each person for something that was characteristic of him or her.

Example: George, would you give me something? I'd like some of your strength. Barbara, would you give me some of your creativity? Another was asked to share his spontaneity, another protection. If you gave me some of your warmth and protection, I could get rid of this cold shield. To his wife, he said: Would you give me some of your anger, some negativity? It's the one thing you withhold from me.

Exercise 38: Expressing Feelings

Break up into groups of threes, choosing the people in the group you know least well. One person will be the monologuer, one the listener, one the recorder. Each member of the threesome will have a turn in each role.

The monologuer begins by telling the listener about his/her initial reactions to the pregnancy and about the way those feelings have been evolving. The listener simply listens without response—either in words, or facial or body response. The listener is present as a nonjudgmental mirror. The recorder makes notes of what is being said so that the speaker has another point of observation to refer to. After about five or ten minutes, the roles are switched until each person has had a chance to be the speaker.

When it has moved around the circle, the threesome can share their reactions and observations with their threesome and later with the group as a whole.

Exercise 39: Nonverbal Hand Conversation

Stand in a circle; hold hands. Stay with your own feelings, yet in touch with each other. Sense each other. Break from the circle and join hands with your spouse. Be with each other nonverbally. Communicate your feelings through your hands. With one hand, shake hands, say hello . . . play . . . Then let the hands fight . . . then let the hands make up . . . be impatient or teasing—and become loving again. . . . Then say good-bye. Share the feelings that were evoked with the group.

Exercise 40: Two Massage Exercises

Massage—Sensing, Exploring, Giving and Taking

Intimacy is central to the experience of pregnancy and birth for both partners. Becoming attuned to each other's needs and feelings through sensing and touching builds a foundation for family times ahead. In the first years, each parent will need to understand the needs of their new baby and be able to express feelings without relying on words.

Giving and receiving through sensitive touching are personal art forms that can enrich every relationship we have. How wonderful it feels to be touched! How much we can understand about another simply through touch. Barriers can be broken through, deep feelings can be expressed, nurturing can occur quite simply.

There are many ways to expand your sensitivity, and some of the books mentioned in the Bibliography will be quite helpful. Here is one exercise from *Your Second Life,* by Gay Gaer Luce, for the group to use in early sessions when they are just getting to know each other. Working with someone less familiar to you can expand your sensitivity to your partner. Move slowly into physical contact, aware of each group member's vulnerable feelings and differences.

Back to Back and Face to Face

Settle on the floor with a partner, either your own or another member of the group. The first time you do the exercise it might be best to do it with the person you know least in the group. When you are sitting comfortably with your back against your partner's back, close your eyes and take a few deep breaths. Begin to feel the rhythm of your partner's breathing. As you get into synchrony with your partner's breathing rhythm, sense what he or she may be feeling. Give yourselves a few minutes to be together in this way.

Next, in turn and without speaking to each other, each of you will become the support for the other. One of you lean back against your partner until your head is resting on your partner's head. Relax your body, especially your shoulders. Just allow your partner to support your weight. As you relax and lean back, your partner will slowly begin to straighten his-her back to be a better supporter.

Now begin to roll your back against your partner's and each of you can massage the back of the other as you move against each other's backs, shoulders, neck and head.

After you have switched so that each partner has had a chance to be both supporter and supported, turn around and face each other. Again in turn, wordlessly and with eyes closed, touch each other's faces and gently explore and massage the forehead, around the eyes, the cheeks, the nose and so forth until all of the face has been explored. Take time and sense what your partner may be feeling and what you are feeling yourself as your hands move over your partner's face.

After each of you has had your turn, open your eyes and share your experience with each other and with the group later if you like.

Massage

One person lies on the floor. All the members of the group gather around the person and massage her or him. You can give them a face, back and shoulder, foot or entire body massage. Be gentle and nurturing, stroking tenderly yet working into tense muscles.

Another way can be for couples to work on each other in turn. It is a very nurturing way to be with each other.

There are some very good books available on massage technique, several of which are listed in the Bibliography.

Exercise 41: Chanting a Name

An exercise for a mother or father who needs loving attention.

Sit in the center of a circle formed by the group and, after looking around at each person in the group that is surrounding you, close your eyes and relax. Focus attention on your breathing rhythm first and, then as you become calm, imagine that you are opening the entire surface of your body to receive the vibration of your name. . . . The group starts to chant your name quietly, allowing the sound to develop as it will. Allow it to continue as long as the group feeling is there and until it ends in a natural way.

The sensory experience of having your name chanted is surprising.

Exercise 42: Affection Bombardment

Several times in the group, after one or another tearfully expressed fear, frustration or distress, we did an exercise called

"Affection Bombardment," a rather simple, obvious and effective group gesture of affection. All of the members of the group surround the person, hold her or him in their arms, cradling, rocking and relaxing. As you can imagine, it is effective and beautiful and the child in each of us needs this sort of loving attention at times.

Exercise 43: Visit to the Doctor—A Role-Playing Exercise

Several members of the group act out a typical visit to the doctor. The mother can watch while someone plays her part. Her partner might choose to do that, or someone else. Someone plays the doctor, someone else the nurse or whatever parts the woman who is directing the activity designates. It should follow the details of her actual experience. After she describes her usual visit, she can replay it, this time asking all the questions she forgot to ask, saying all the things she meant to say or was afraid to say. It can be rehearsed several times until she feels clear about her needs. Repetition usually reveals hidden agendas and also increases self-confidence. Fathers can also participate in the same way.

Exercise 44: Rehearsal for Birth

Start with a relaxation exercise. Then with eyes closed, focus on the word *birth*. Allow whatever images, words or feelings to arise. . . . It is the time for the baby to be born. . . . Imagine how the birth might take place. How would you like it to be—for you and for your baby? Visualize the physical place, the people who will be there, the ambience. . . . Where are you? Who is with you? What are they doing? Let the drama unfold. You are the producer-director. It may be a symbol, a whole scenario, a fleeting image. Accept what comes. It will develop in your unconscious and continue to emerge perhaps later in a dream or a waking fantasy—trust your unconscious to work it through.

When you feel satisfied with what is happening in your fantasy, come slowly back to this room and this moment. . . . Tell your partner what you envisioned and then share with the group.

This exercise can be practiced several times before the birth. Your capacity to imagine what you want will develop progressively each time. You can write your image, draw it or speak it into a tape recorder.

Exercise 45: Welcoming the Baby

The baby is at the center of this transformation that is taking place. This exercise can be used over and over with different feelings evoked each time, I'm sure.

Lie down. Close your eyes and relax in whatever way feels good for you. Take time to unwind and let go. Don't rush into the second part of the exercise until you feel that each part of your body has let go of its tension. Check through your whole body slowly. Are you now relaxed?

Begin to smile, still with your eyes closed. Sense what happens to your mouth as you smile, as your lips elongate, as your cheek muscles tighten to create a smile. Sense all the small changes that occur in your face as your smile gets larger.

How do you feel as you smile? What happens to the rest of your face? And your shoulders and your spine? Move through your body and invite it to participate in the smile. How does that happen for you?

Now, when you feel that your whole being is smiling, envision the baby. Mothers, put your hands over the womb. Fathers, become part of the triangle in whatever way feels comfortable.

When you feel that you are in touch with the baby and that your breathing rhythms are coordinated, communicate your pleasure to the baby and tell it what you are feeling about its arrival. Try to transfer all the good feelings that accompany your smiling person to your baby. Tell it how welcome it is and will be.

IX:

The Environment of Birth—Visions of a Family-Centered Birth House

The nest house is . . . the natural habitat of the function of inhabiting. For not only do we come back to it, but we dream of coming back to it, the way a bird comes back to its nest, or a lamb to its fold. This sign of return marks an infinite number of daydreams, for the reason that human returning takes place in the great rhythm of human life, a rhythm that reaches back across the years and, through the dream, combats all absence.

In this domain, everything takes place simply and delicately.

Gaston Bachelard,
The Poetics of Space

First: What *is* environment?

Environment is what surrounds us, and affects and influences our growth and development. It is:

- the complex web of psychological, social, cultural, ecological and transpersonal conditions that form us;
- the envelope we call our body, its form and shape and its biology;
- our culture influencing and altering our biology;
- our body expressing who we are, how we feel, how we wish to be seen and experienced;
- our mind organizing the sensory input our bodies receive from the external world;
- the language we share and personalize.

It includes our myths, our fears, our love, our connection to each other . . . and our inherited and unique experiences, as the human species, as individuals . . . an unending spiral that we only partially perceive and which affects our every turn.

During the course of the many transitions we make in a day, we move in and out of many environments. Many of these transitions are mundane and ordinary: I wake up from a dream state, tumble out of bed and move through the cooler air of the hallway into the bathroom. It is the first of many multitransitions through which I will pass in the course of the day. My miniature environments change and yet are interconnected. Many are chosen by me, are in fact extensions of myself which give particular definition to my life: my house, my car, my neighborhood, my favorite restaurant or market. Other environments are less personal: the street, an office, public transportation. They may be constricting, ugly and exhausting; others may be harmonious, beautiful, nurturing. I cope with all of these more or less unconsciously. They are part of my ordinary daily experience and integrally affect the way I feel and behave.

Some environments are extraordinary, like Chartres Cathedral, or the Grand Canyon, or our very first environment—the womb. Some transitions are singular, monumental, like our very first transition—birth.

The development of the baby in the extraordinary environment of the womb has become for me a primary example of the interconnectedness, interdependence and interpenetration of all things. In that remarkably designed, bounded and protected environment, we pass through many subtle transitory stages. And perhaps each time we make a major transition in our lives, and move from a known experience to an unknown one, we may be reflecting some aspect of our first transition. This first environment and these primal transitions may indeed be the template for later ones. It seems simple and obvious that we should design the first transition to be as nurturing and harmonious as possible so that it becomes a positive base for future transitions.

So much has happened in the past decade to make us more aware of birth. The deepening of consciousness that began in the '60s and the integration of that awareness into action-oriented programs of the '70s and '80s have been partly responsible. The resurgence of interest in home births, in both rural and urban areas, has deeply influenced attitudes among parents and health care professionals around the country. The increasing cost of a traditional hospital delivery has had something to do with the changes, too. With a declining birth rate, doctors and hospitals have wanted to attract expectant parents to their institutions and have altered practices to meet consumer demands. New research on the effects of using drugs and bonding is being taken into account in some places, though often the changes and the importance of infant-mother bonding being made are experimental and limited. Mt. Zion Hospital in San Francisco now offers a bedroom-like "alternative birth suite" with a minimum of medical equipment and an attractive homelike birthing room, as do many others now across the country. A most important element in this environment is the quality, tenderness and supportiveness of the medical staff. This new design occurred as a result of the personal delivery experience of the chief of pediatrics in the hospital. When she was having her own baby, she was appalled at how inhumane, threatening and "insensitive" the environment was.

Other models of alternative birth environments are emerging. Some are fortunate enough to have financial support in their home states, like the new birth center being planned in Taos, New Mexico. In Menlo Park and San Jose, California, two limited-capacity out-of-hospital centers opened in the fall of 1979 with the ultimate goal of providing the full range of support services to make alternative birth practices available to everyone. Assemblyman John Vasconcelles has introduced legislation to ease current restrictions and permit these explorative models to prove their validity.

An important bill that has been put into effect by Vasconcelles is one that establishes a commission to seek out the root causes of violence in our society. Possible long-term effects of birthing practices are some of the main areas to be examined. Guidelines are being proposed for training lay midwives, and resource guides have been developed: *Resource Guide on Alternative Birthing in California* (Cougar Books, P.O. Box 22246, Scaramento, Calif. 95822). Most important, medical malpractice insurance coverage has been obtained for the two California centers. The right to obtain routine insurance coverage for the costs of births must now also be granted, so that services can be available to all who want them. Although these two centers can by no means fill the demand for an alternative birth environment, they may serve as a model for other communities on the West Coast. Individuals in other parts of the country have been working toward these changes for a long time. These efforts date from the turn of the century; for example, the work of the Chicago Maternity Center in the early 1900s, the Frontier Nursing Service in Kentucky in the '20s, and the Maternity Center Association in New York City. Over thirty years ago, it was at the Maternity Center that I prepared for the births of my three children. In the 1940s, they were training nurse-midwives in New York City and introduced Grantley Dick-Read's methods and ideas to the United States. Ruth Lubec, Director of the Maternity Center, has continued to pioneer new alternatives and recently opened a clinic for nurse-midwife attended births within seven minutes of a hospital in New York City. Yet, sadly, despite their excellent track record as a responsible innovative force, their center's existence is constantly under attack. Perhaps in the 1980s we will finally win widespread acceptance of our right to have safe, supervised nonhospital births.

Clearly, in the past decade, we have been witnessing a revolution in attitudes toward nature, toward health and toward the management of birth. Women—and men—want to reown their bodies, minds and feelings.

Over lunch with English author and childbirth educator Sheila Kitzinger, I questioned why the alternative birth movement was happening now. Kitzinger replied,

> It seems there comes a time when people can hear. The great propagandists are ones who understand timing and don't say more than people can hear at a given moment. It seems extraordinary to me that people are able to now hear the very same words that were being spoken for many long years. In order to present an idea, it has to be bold and simple. I think that's what Leboyer has done by focusing a strong light on one particular area and one defined moment in human experience.

Leboyer's poetic and humane message has affected men and women. Yet, despite all the new information that has accumulated, and the increased availability of childbirth preparation classes, women who are pregnant for the first time are still as excited *and* as uncertain as any woman has been since the beginning of time. Women and men still have to discover all the complexities of the pregnant state for themselves. This knowledge doesn't seem to be accessible on a conscious level before pregnancy and there is little in our education to prepare us. Unlike other transitions in our lives, giving birth and becoming parents isn't a passage that we consider very much until its actuality and immediacy is upon us.

Actually, the care and psychological nurturance of pregnant parents needs to be considered the social responsibility of the culture and to become an integral part of a prenatal mental health program funded by the government. Indeed, we all have a responsibility to the next generation. How each parent deals with this rite of passage depends not only on his or her unique personal history, but also on our shared cultural history. We need to offer new healthy ways for *people* to make the transition into parenthood.

Man, woman, child—each one of us is deeply involved with this experience of coming into being and birth. We come at it every which way—scientifically, spiritually, mystically, intuitively. The way we view it will affect the way we manage the process and the way we behave and the way the baby will develop in the womb.

How can we make the transfer of experience and insight a more natural one, so that there is less discontinuity between the pregnant and nonpregnant state? How can we all be enriched by the insight and expanded consciousness that this experience provides? How can we create supportive rituals and patterns that allow us to gain from the far-reaching dimensions of this rite of passage? Lots of questions. Some answers from me. Others must come from you. Collaborative effort will bring us closer to solutions.

I am now aware of some of these dimensions. How can I and others like me best make available what we know and feel?

It is clear to me that we need to create holistic birth centers which would incorporate old ideas and new ones, weaving together the strands of intuition and knowledge.

In this chapter, I offer my vision of such a holistic, family-centered environment for birth.

Why a Holistic Birth Center?

When I visited many years ago with A. S. Neill, author of *Summerhill* and headmaster of an innovative nontraditional English school, he related this story about one of the small children in his school who, in a fight with a classmate, hurt his hand rather badly. When the school nurse examined it, she decided that it required hospital care. As she set out to drive the boy to the local hospital, he insisted on seeing Neill first. "What can I do for you that the nurse can't do?" asked Neill of the teary boy, who insisted that Neill drive him to the hospital. The small boy looked up at the six-foot-tall Scotsman with love and trust and said, "She'll take care of my hand, but you'll take care of all of me."

This same attitude and approach is accepted as a guideline in holistic medicine. It has come to mean an approach to health that takes into account the whole person and not only his-her illness, but the integration of mind, body, spirit, viewing the person instead in relation to the entire context in which he-she lives—the family, the social and cultural milieu, the environment. It sees people from the point of view of health rather than illness and encourages the patient to participate in the healing process in an active and informed way. Holistic approaches include many nontraditional healing practices which have been ignored in Western medicine until recently.

A thousand years ago, the Chinese organized prenatal clinics to guide a woman through pregnancy, believing that her emotions and biology together influenced the nature and future behavior and mental health of her child. Consequently, the culture fostered her emotional tranquillity, as well as her physical well-being. We, too, need a place that concerns itself not only with our bodies but also with our psyche and spirit.

We need to create holistic environments where expectant parents are cared for and supported during this rite of passage. Environments that help them practice life as an art, while they are involved with the very essence of being—the creation of a new person. We need to provide opportunities for them to explore themselves, to "loosen the knots," to reassess their life as they prepare for parenthood—environments in which they begin to understand what governs their choices. Birth centers would enable expectant parents to celebrate the transformation taking place instead of "laboring" through the transition. We need environments in which everything important about birth could be discussed, acted on and evaluated during the entire childbearing year.

Basic questions underlie one's considerations in designing such a center.

What is a holistic attitude?

How does a point of view get stated in spatial terms, or physical environments? And then affect behavior and double back on itself? How do we view birth? And how will we change our views?

Many questions need to be asked by everyone involved: parents, health professionals, social scientists, foundations distributing funds, insurance companies, government agencies, medical associations—all those involved with the delivery and regulation of health care needed by expectant parents.

What could a modern birth center offer to a couple either before or after they conceived?

Imagine if parents could come to the center just to consider whether or not they wanted to have a baby, if they had others to talk with as they worked through their ambivalent feelings about becoming parents—others who might be skilled counselors or parents who were further along on the parenting journey—just as Alan and Rachel did. They might have a chance to cuddle a friend's drowsy, sweet-smelling infant or try to quiet a wet, cranky toddler as they all talked, just as young people used to in smaller, more intimate communities when life was simpler and families and friends were closer and more involved in each other's lives. They might then be able to make plans with more emotional clarity. By loosening the psyche's knots even before conception, they might be ready to participate more fully and bring to that creative moment of conception a level of clarity of consciousness and deep love that would transfer itself to the person coming into life. How different is the act when a child is conceived out of love and is invited, as it were, to come into being? How might the atmosphere of love be felt by the developing organism? We know that stress is communicated to the baby—why not love? The mystics have long talked of this.

The environment of the birth center would cater to the pregnant year—to all the aspects of preparenting, birth and the first few postpartum months, giving support to the emergent family as it progressed through its growing pains. It would be planned so that it included the three-generational family, and surrogate families as well, for we know that this passage affects siblings, grandparents and other members of the family, indirectly, in important ways. So far removed are we these days from an integrated view of family life that we tend to overlook the effects on all those involved.

A birth center could provide an environment where there is continuity of experience with other expectant parents and with a professional staff who will serve as knowledgeable guides throughout the entire period. The staff would be sensitive to the emotional well-being of the couple, as well as to the physical aspects of giving birth. It would be a place where people communicate with the heart as well as the intellect, where grace is taught in the womb—a place where parents could practice listening to their own innate wisdom and can honor their extraordinary state of consciousness. Together, the parents and their health team could meet and come to know each other as they embark on this journey. Together, they would reach decisions that reflected the parents' values and life design rather than asking parents to fit into institutionalized choices, methods and routines. Parents would therefore participate in their own evolution and the evolution of the center as well. It would be an environment in which, with the help of professional staff, parents could learn about their bodies and psyches. It would be a place in which they could share the responsibility for their own health and well-being and participate in their own care. Obviously, no one wants to go back in time and give up modern medical advances that are beneficial and have cut down mortality for mother and child; however, a normal pregnancy should not be treated as an illness. Birth centers do not mock medical advances; rather, they make use of our increased scientific knowledge to enhance the experience—as background instead of foreground. It is important that the ambience of the center project a sense of order; it should strive to reduce uncertainty, feel familiar and safe, be enfolding and tranquil.

It would be a place in which parents can create new personal rituals out of shared experience.

Design of the Center

The practical aspects of the services at the center might be divided into four stages—preconception, pregnancy, delivery and postnatal—each characterized by both unique and interrelated concerns. At each stage, three levels of the experience would be considered: intrapersonal (our inner selves), interpersonal (communication with others), transpersonal (beyond the boundaries of our own egos—the universal dimension).

The center would be designed to reflect the symbolic and specific aspects of the lives of the individuals in the group it serves. In some cultures, these important passages are celebrated with others around; in others, quite privately. It is important to honor these roots. We know that unconscious levels of the psyche are activated during this period. In fact, it may be one of the most significant aspects of the experience that leads to further growth.

One of the most relevant arguments for home birth is the

familiarity of the setting. At home, all the subtle patterns are comfortable, known. There need be no unconscious search for recognizable symbols; they have already been created and accepted. When so much change is taking place, dealing with unfamiliar people, rules and physical space is an added stress. A doctor friend said, "Putting a couple in a strange hospital room and asking the woman to give birth is like asking a couple to make love while we watch." A birth center which has already become incorporated into one's psyche as a known and familiar environment can be a source of comfort and support.

Each environment has a message. Its voice is as clear as the verbal message of the person who receives the parents as they enter the center. Parents, in their uniquely vulnerable state, will be as sensitive to its ambience as is photographic paper when exposed to the light.

In a warm enveloping physical setting, staffed with affirming, knowing guides—teachers, doctors, nurse-midwives, psychologists and others—we would offer prenatal education and care, films, lectures and workshops.

Heterogeneous groups of couples and single parents at different stages of pregnancy would explore together their ordinary everyday feelings along with the extraordinary and the less-examined aspects of pregnancy. They would be able to focus on all aspects of the developing relationship of the mother and the father and the unborn child. The following chart suggests some of the attributes of my ideal birth center.

What would be available to a couple who came to such a center?

The birth center would be a facility for prenatal care, delivery and birth, and postnatal care of the largest proportion of women giving birth—those who expect a normal, uncomplicated pregnancy and birth. Preventive care and early detection of existing and potential problems would be part of the program. Proper screening must take place, of course, to make sure that all mothers are indeed low-risk, and precautionary measures would be available for the unforeseen emergencies both at the center and at a backup hospital which would be no more than seven to ten minutes away.

Psychological (Counseling)

- Counseling with professionals
- Self-led groups
- Prepregnant groups
- Pregnancy groups
- Individual and couple therapy
- Postnatal groups
- Infant psychology

Physiological (Medical)

- Prenatal education
- Prenatal care—check-ups
- Nutritional—exercise information
- Midwife consultation—physician consultation
- Prepared childbirth techniques—methods of all kinds
- Breastfeeding information
- Infant care
- Training program for physicians, midwives, psychologists

Physical Space (Environment)

- Reception room with welcoming symbolic entry
- Kitchen for waiting, meeting, gathering, eating
- Garden for conversing, sitting contemplatively, strolling, planting, waiting
- Examination room and bathrooms
- Clinical lab
- Emergency rooms
- Meeting rooms for mind-body practices, yoga, meditation, biofeedback, breathing practices, massage, water therapy
- Staff room
- Music room for listening, making music

- Reference library—books, records, films, periodicals
- Thrift shop for maternity and infant clothes and furniture
- Three to six birth rooms reached by a separate entrance through the garden—double beds, extra bed for partner or coach

To facilitate the process of "loosening the knots" during the pregnant year, we would use many ways of exploring consciousness that have been developed in Eastern philosophy and by the human potential movement, techniques like Gestalt, psychodrama, transactional analysis; body techniques that involve movement, sound and massage; methods of meditation, psychosynthesis and dream therapies. Keeping journals would be encouraged as a creative way of recording poems and drawings and understanding dreams and fantasies.

Various techniques would be taught, to ease the tension and pain that can develop during labor and delivery; these would include meditation, hypnosis, biofeedback training, breath control techniques like those of hatha yoga and kundalini yoga and sound anesthesia like chants, mantras and music. Also available would be the traditional methods taught by Lamaze, Kitzinger, Bradley and others.

Imagine a center that would be either in the city, overlooking a park, or outside the center of the city, close to water, woods or mountains and yet within minutes of a hospital. . . .

Whether in the city, the suburbs or the country, it would be a space flooded with the light that is so essential to growing things. Imagine an airy pavilion of loosely connected rooms surrounding a garden. . . . The entrance door would be reached through a passage covered with a bower of flowering vines. This rite of passage is symbolically expressed in the design of the entrance—the way in and out—a metaphor so particular to conception and birth. If, as Carl Jung suggests, the house is the symbol of the self beyond the body, we see the need for the birth house to express a poetic consciousness of what this transformation is about in spatial form. This place—this physical space—can become a calm, secure, protective environment for parents-to-be as they cross the threshold into parenthood.

* * *

Every threshold crossed marks a new state, every door
entered a step forward in constant renewal, where the
wheel of life expands and contracts, following the universal
spiral, leading humanity from inside to outside, from
periphery to center, in a rhythm inexorably tied to that of
the planets and the atom.

> Olivier, Marc,
> *The Psychology of the House*

As one moves across the threshold and through the portal,
there is a welcoming central reception room which in turn opens
into a garden which can be seen through the glassy walls.

The garden is central to the plan. In it I envision a large tree
with low, spreading limbs—a tree of life. A tree to sit in and
under—an enveloping organic reminder of the changing seasons,
and the processes of regeneration and birth.

I see the garden filled with life—abounding with the colors,
smells, sounds, rhythms and movement of living things: birds,
small animals, flowering plants, moving water, fertile earth. The
care and growth of the garden would reflect and affirm a similar
process taking place for the parents as the pregnancy unfolds. It
would have the simplicity and tranquillity of a Japanese garden,
which symbolizes the elements of the entire universe, with its
rocks, water, trees, earth.

In many cultures, a tree planting ceremony is customary: in
Switzerland, it is an apple tree for a boy, a pear tree for a girl; in
Haiti, a coconut tree for both. Recently, some young friends of
mine in Massachusetts created this ceremony after the birth of
their first child. The mother happened to be an anthropologist:

> For Peter, who was born three days ago: We buried your
> placenta and planted a tree above it to represent your
> connection with the earth and all of life. Next to it, we
> buried a peach, an apple and a plum, symbolizing you,
> the fruit of my womb and the seed of our lives.

* * *

You might create your own personal ceremony. Can you imagine a more beautiful way to reforest the earth?

The garden would serve as a place to talk with others, to read, or simply to be alone in contemplative silence—a place to sense one's own rhythms and the rhythm of the universe to which each of us is attuned.

Woven into the fabrics of the furnishings and decorating the walls would be birth symbols and images from all over the world to nourish our intuitive understanding of the designs and artifacts that symbolize the universal mystery, magic and miracle of birth.

Rooms would be homelike and large enough to accommodate family or friends. Ideally, each room would have a shower, toilet and a washbasin. It would be wonderful if rooms opened onto balconies overlooking the garden.

Making furnishings for the center might be part of the activity of the workshops: weaving or painting or creating a joint wall hanging in the manner of the old-fashioned wedding quilts, with birth symbols used instead. Textures of wool, straw, reed and pottery would mirror the organic nature of the gestation and birth process. Particular consideration would be given to the healing qualities of color, sound and light, and the tactile sense of materials—to the psychological effects of the sensory environment. For example, sound is used in various cultures during labor and delivery: music by the Laotians of Southeast Asia, the Navajo Indians and the Cuna Indians of Panama; and conversation as pure sound stimulation to ease birth pain by many tribes who pattern delivery as a social event. Sontag's research, as we have seen in Chapter II, demonstrates that sound affects both the mother and the unborn child.

Earth colors might prevail: warm embracing combinations of golden yellows, pomegranate reds, persimmon oranges accented by indigo and sky-blues, plum-purples and the leaf-greens of springtime.

Soft downy-cushioned chairs and couches would enfold one.

Comfortable flexible seating arrangements would invite all kinds of exchange in both group and private consultation and promote informal conversation and friendship. Close by the sitting room, a large kitchen would provide a family atmosphere in which people might gather at a circular wooden table for food or coffee near a warming fire. In this nurturing environment, food, feelings, knowledge and experience would be shared. Extended family support systems could develop quite naturally. Kitchen table consultation could take place informally with staff, about everything from nutrition to treatment of simple ailments and the demands of the emerging family. Exchange about the most intimate and urgent concerns might take place among the parents quite casually over coffee.

Other rooms that serve particular functions would surround the atrium. Consultation and examining rooms, designed in a warm, nonclinical fashion, would contain the necessary medical and technical equipment and would encourage trusting, self-responsible interactions between staff and clients. Rooms for group meetings and for various body therapies—for massage, saunas and mineral baths—would be available for healthy exercise, pleasure and sensory expansion: spaces for group work, for dancing, for yoga, for meditation. New aids, such as biofeedback training, found to be helpful for relaxation and for teaching about one's inner states would also be available, as would a library filled with the newest books, periodicals, records, films, slides about childbirth and parenting, self-care and self-awareness, and a music room for listening to and making music.

Lighting in the rooms would be controlled by dimmers which allow parents and medical staff to select the level of light during labor. Chairs and beds would be designed for comfort and flexibility and facilitation of labor and delivery. Double beds would accommodate fathers and mothers and perhaps the smaller children in the family—parents would bring personal mementos—a musical instrument or record, game or a piece of art to meditate on—whatever would give comfort and feel more like home, just as the couple in my group did:

* * *

We took a lot of things from home like a book of poetry, a quilt (which we never used but it made us feel good to have it folded on a chair and available)and favorite records.

New architectural forms could be used for the center, inspired by the shapes that the animal world uses to build its nests, cocoons and shelters. Or by the shapes of the earliest dwellings of man, such as caves. Shelters that reiterate womb shapes. We might choose circular dwellings such as are used by many societies that live in close harmony with their natural environment: the igloos of the Eskimos, the wigwams of the Indians, the *kraals* of the African tribes and the *yurts* of the Mongols. Or the contemporary geodesic dome of Buckminster Fuller, or the sculptured shapes of Paoli Soleri in Arizona, which also harmoniously invite the interaction of man and nature. The spherical configuration of a dome attunes us to the celestial environment, to the rising and setting sun, to the phases of the moon, solstices and equinoxes.

Imagine giving birth under the stars and the light of the full moon.

Imagine a dome that unfolds like a lotus, opening to the warm breezes of the spring, summer or fall sky.

The aperture, "the eye of the dome," as Mircea Eliade puts it, "has classically symbolized breakthrough from plane to plane, communication with the transcendent." Childbirth itself is such an opening.

This dream of childbearing opens up the possibilities of an alternate reality for the pregnant year. I am reminded of the teaching of the Senoi tribe in Malaysia, who ask their children when they have a nightmare to sleep again and recreate a less frightening scenario in order to repattern their behavior and experience. Similarly, there is creative potential in a positive dream of childbirth. Let us create a vision of the possible.

Let us create an environment for the pregnant year and birth that reflects the glory and mystery of being human.

Bibliography

General

Castaneda, Carlos. *Journey to Ixtlan: The Lessons of Don Juan.* New York: Simon and Schuster, 1972.

———*A Separate Reality: Further Conversations with Don Juan.* New York: Simon and Schuster, A Touchstone Book, 1971.

———*The Teachings of Don Juan: A Yaqui Way of Knowledge.* Berkeley and Los Angeles: University of California Press, 1968.

Firestone, Shulamith. *The Dialectic of Sex.* New York: William Morrow and Co., 1970.

Fodor, Nandor. *The Search for the Beloved.* New York: University Books, 1969.

Fromm, Erich. *The Art of Loving.* New York: Harper & Row Pub., Inc., 1974.

Grof, Stanislav. *Realms of the Human Unconscious.* New York. Viking Press, 1975.

Harding, M. Esther. *Women's Mysteries.* New York: Putnam, C. J. Jung Foundation Series, 1971.

Laing, R. D. *The Politics of the Family.* New York: Pantheon Books, 1971.

————*The Facts of Life.* New York: Pantheon Books, 1976.

Lang, Raven. *Birth Book.* Palo Alto, Calif.: Genesis Press, 1972.

Leboyer, Frederick. *Birth Without Violence.* New York: Alfred A. Knopf, 1975.

————*Loving Hands.* New York: Alfred A. Knopf, 1976.

Maslow, Abraham H. *Toward a Psychology of Being.* New York: Van Nostrand Reinhold, 1968.

May, Rollo. *Love and Will.* New York: W. W. Norton & Co., Inc., 1969.

Mead, Margaret. *Male and Female.* New York: Wm. Morrow, 1975.

Newman, E. *The Great Mother.* New York: Pantheon Books, 1955.

Nilsson, Lennart. *Behold Man.* Boston: Little, Brown and Co., 1973.

Olivier, Marc. *The Psychology of the House.* New York: Thames and Hudson, 1977.

————*Resource Guide on Alternative Birthing in California.* Sacramento, Calif.: Cougar Books, 1980.

Rank, Otto. *The Trauma of Birth.* New York: Harper/Torch-books, 1973.

Suzuki, Shunryu. *Zen Mind, Beginner's Mind.* New York: John Weatherhill, Inc., 1970.

Prenatal/Postnatal Emotions

Bittman, Sam, and Sue Zalk. *Expectant Fathers.* New York: Hawthorn Books, 1978.

Colman, Arthur D., and Libby L. Colman. *Pregnancy: The Psychological Experience.* New York: Seabury Press, 1971.

Deutsch, Helene. *The Psychology of Women.* London: Research Books, Ltd., 1947.

Meltzer, David. *Birth.* New York: Ballantine Books, 1973.

Montagu, Ashley. *Touching: The Human Significance of Skin.* New York: Wiley, 1964.

Newton, Niles. *Maternal Emotions.* New York: Paul B. Hoeber, Inc., 1963.

Biological Aspects of Pregnancy and Birth

American College of Obstetricians and Gynecologists. *Family-centered Maternity/Newborn Care in Hospitals.* One E. Wacker Drive, Suite 270, Chicago, Illinois 60601.

Arms, Suzanne. *Immaculate Deception.* Boston: Houghton Mifflin Co., 1975.

Boston Women's Health Book Collective. *Ourselves and Our Children.* New York: Random House, 1978.

Bradley, Robert A. *Husband-Coached Childbirth.* New York: Harper & Row Pub., Inc., 1974.

Brook, Danae. *Naturbirth.* New York: Pantheon Books, 1976.

Flanagan, Geraldine. *The First Nine Months of Life.* New York: Simon and Schuster, 1962.

Hotchner, Tracy. *Pregnancy and Childbirth.* New York: Avon, 1979.

Howells, John, ed. *Modern Perspectives in Psycho-obstetrics.* New York: Brunner-Mazel, 1972.

Kitzinger, Sheila. *The Experience of Childbirth.* New York: Penguin, 1967.

Meltzer, David. *Birth.* New York: Ballantine Books, 1973.

Milinaire, Caterine. *Birth.* New York: Harmony Books, 1971.

Montagu, Ashley. *Life Before Birth.* New York: New American Library, 1964.

Nilsson, Lennart; Axel Ingelman, et al. *A Child Is Born.* New York: Dell, 1969.

Petty, Roy. *Home Birth: A Complete Authoritative Guide to the*

Back-to-Basics Trend in Childbirth. Northbrook, Illinois: Domus Books.

Rosen, Mortimer G., and Lynn Rosen. *Your Baby's Brain Before Birth.* New York: New American Library, 1975.

Rugh, Roberts and Landrum Shettles. *From Conception to Birth: The Drama of Life's Beginnings.* New York: Harper & Row Pub., Inc., 1971.

Creative Sex During Pregnancy

Bing, Elisabeth and Libby Colman. *Making Love During Pregnancy.* New York: Bantam Books, 1977.

Comfort, Alex. *The Joy of Sex.* New York: Crown Publishers, 1972.

Gillico, Jerry. *Transcendental Sex: A Meditational Approach to Increasing Sensual Pleasure.* Toronto: Holt, Rinehart & Winston, 1978.

Awareness Exercises

Anderson, Marianne S., and Louis M. Savary. *Passages: A Guide for Pilgrims of the Mind.* New York: Harper & Row Pub., Inc., 1972.

Assagioli, Roberto. *Psychosynthesis.* New York: Viking/Compass, 1965.

Berne, Eric. *Games People Play.* New York: Grove Press, 1969.

Bonny, Helen, and Louis Savary. *Music and Your Mind.* New York: Harper & Row Pub., Inc., 1973.

Brooks, Charles V.W. *Sensory Awareness: The Rediscovery of Experiencing.* New York: Viking Press, 1974.

Carter, Mildred. *Helping Yourself with Foot Reflexology*. Englewood Cliffs, New Jersey: Parker Publishing Co., 1969.

Delancey, Gayle. *Living Your Dreams*. New York: Harper & Row Pub., Inc., 1979.

Downing, George. *The Massage Book*. New York: Random House, 1970; Random House/Bookworks, 1974.

Faraday, Ann. *Dream Power*. New York: Coward, McCann, 1972.

Garfield, Patricia. *Creative Dreaming*. New York: Simon and Schuster, 1975.

Grossman, Richard. *Choosing and Changing*. New York: E.P. Dutton, 1978.

Gunther, Bernard. *Sense Relaxation*. New York: Collier Books, 1968.

Hills, Christopher, and Deborah Rozman. *Exploring Inner Space: Awareness Games for All Ages*. Boulder Creek, California: University of Trees, 1978.

Jacobson, Edmund. *Progressive Relaxation*. Chicago: University of Chicago Press, 1974.

———*How to Relax and Have Your Baby*. New York: McGraw Hill, 1959.

Keyes, Margaret F. *The Inward Journey: Art as Therapy for You*. Millbrae, California: Celestial Arts, 1974.

Leedy, Jack J. *Poetry, the Healer*. New York: Lippincott, 1973.

Lewis, Howard R., and Dr. Harold S. Streitfeld. *Growth Games*. New York: Harcourt Brace Jovanovich, 1970.

Luce, Gary Gaer. *Your Second Life*. New York: Delacorte Press, Seymour Lawrence, 1979.

Masters, Robert, and Jean Houston. *Mind Games*. New York: Dell Books, 1972.

Perls, Fritz, M.D., Ph.D. *Gestalt Therapy Verbatim*. Lafayette, California: Real People Press, 1969.

Perls, Fritz, R. Hefferline and P. Goodman. *Gestalt Therapy*. New York: Delta Books, 1951.

Progoff, Ira. *At a Journal Workshop*. New York: Dialogue House Library, 1975.

Rhyne, Janie. *The Gestalt Art Experience.* Monterey, California: Brooks/Cole, 1973.

Rogers, Carl R. *On Becoming a Person.* Boston: Houghton Mifflin, 1961.

———*On Encounter Groups.* New York: Harper & Row Pub., Inc., 1970.

———*On Personal Power.* New York: Delacorte, 1977.

Samuels, Mike, and Nancy Samuels. *Seeing with the Mind's Eye.* New York: Random House/Bookworks, 1975.

Satir, Virginia. *Peoplemaking.* California: Science & Behavior Books, 1972.

Schultz, William C. *Joy.* New York: Grove Press, 1967.

Simon, Sid. *Caring, Feeling, Touching.* Niles, Illinois: Argus, 1976.

Smith, David. *The East-West Exercise Book.* New York: McGraw Hill, 1976.

Stevens, John O. *Awareness: Exploring, Experimenting, Experiencing.* New York: Bantam Books, 1973.

Trungpa, Chogyam. *Dharmas Without Blame.* Berkeley, California: Shambala Publications, 1973.

Tulku, Tarthang. *Gesture of Balance: A Guide to Awareness, Self-healing and Meditation.* Emeryville, California: Dharma Publishing, 1977.

———*Time, Space and Knowledge: A New Vision of Reality.* Emeryville, California: Dharma Publishing, 1977.

Vaughn, Frances E. *Awakening Intuition.* New York: Anchor Books, 1979.

White, John, and James Fadiman, eds. *Relax: How You Can Feel Better.* New York: Dell, 1976.

Index